THE P.I.N.K. PRIMER

For

Partners In Need of Koaching

Robert Musser

This book provides general information on how to support a loved one with a serious ill-ness that is based solely on the personal experience of the author. This information should not be used for diagnosis, treatment, or as a substitute for professional medical services. A health care provider should be consulted prior to any treatment or self-care.

Internet addresses provided in this book were accurate at the time it went to press.

Cover Design: Judi Loscomb, Laser Letters, Inc.

First published by Dog Ear Publishing
4010 W. 86th Street, Ste H
Indianapolis, IN 46268
www.dogearpublishing.net

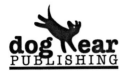

ISBN: 978-160844-176-1

This book is printed on acid-free paper.

Printed in the United States of America

This book is dedicated to all our family and friends who supported us in our journey with breast cancer. A special thank you goes to Dawna Markova and Patty Dean. Their encouragement and direction were invaluable to the publishing of this book.

One in eight women in the United States will develop breast cancer at some point in her life. A significant portion of proceeds from the sale of this book will be donated to organizations supporting women touched by this disease.

Table of Contents

Foreword

I'm not sure how many women write the foreword to their husbands' books, but I don't really care. My husband, Bob, wrote this book to chronicle the breast cancer journey we shared, so I feel I should say something about it.

Bob originally intended the book to be targeted to men who have significant others with breast cancer. He quickly realized that much of the content was applicable to men and women supporting individuals with any type of cancer. This was reinforced during the writing process when his friend David called for advice on how to support his wife battling lung cancer. David and his grown children read the unfinished manuscript and found it immensely useful.

Bob is an opinionated guy who will gladly share his thoughts on most any subject, so he could have written volumes, but that wasn't the intent. His goal was to provide something short and to the point, like CliffsNotes on breast cancer. As a husband, partner, friend and father, Bob wanted to jump into action when I was diagnosed. He wanted to put his best effort forward and figured other men had the same need for their own loved ones.

Piles of information came flying at me, starting the day I was told I had the big BC. Strangely enough, Bob wasn't provided any specific partner support resources. Long after the worst of my battle was over, we discovered that a couple of breast cancer support books for men do exist, but even the medical team we worked with didn't mention them. This is a strange and troubling inconsistency since one in eight women is diagnosed with breast cancer, and each one needs support.

Publishers told us that men don't buy self-help books. This came as no surprise to us given the different socialization process boys and girls go through growing up. For example (and I'm stereotyping here), men don't like to stop and ask for directions when they are lost. They probably learn this from their fathers. Bob readily admits he acts like he knows a lot more about a wide array of subjects than he really does. He says this was how he was brought up—bluff your way through it and figure it out later. Young boys are also taught that guys don't cry, at least not publicly. These aren't bad things and, at times, have served Bob well. But when dealing with breast cancer, it's an entirely different situation. You don't just make it up. You both have to stop and ask questions. We found that talking about feelings is an important part of recovery for men and women.

I am so proud of my partner in life for undertaking this project. Bob has always been a natural writer, but with a career in a totally different area, sitting down to author a book was not on his agenda. Breast cancer changed that. He felt a need to share what we'd learned. It was also a way for Bob to digest what had happened between us when dealing with a life-threatening illness.

You'll get to know my husband in the pages that follow and understand why I so love this funny, quirky guy who makes me smile every day. Enjoy!

E. Ann Musser
Oxford, Maryland

CHAPTER 1

Introduction

The P.I.N.K. Primer...catchy title...pink being the symbolic color for women having breast cancer. In this case however, PINK also stands for "Partners In Need of Koaching." Obviously a misspelling, but what are you going to do?

Now, there is a tremendous amount of literature available to breast cancer patients, but little focuses on how to support those so afflicted. This primer is from a male perspective, although it applies to partners of either sex. So, don't take offense when I use words like "guys." *The P.I.N.K. Primer* has practical guidance for all partners taking this journey with their loved one. In fact, even though I focus on breast cancer, much of the advice offered applies equally to partners supporting a loved one with any type of cancer.

Breast cancer is not a day trip. So, to all my "rat killing" friends, you can just suck it up and get over it! Guys just love to nuke problems, take care of issues, and then put the damned thing to bed and move on. Hey, it's what we do and how we were trained. However, in this case, if you just expand your time horizon, it is doable, though frustrating.

In some respects, this is a story about you and what you do. But it ain't about you! It's about someone you love who means the world to you. Your mission is to keep them around...if you only want to go through the motions, then put this down and grab your remote.

Ill equipped? No kidding, who isn't? Willing to give it your best? Okay, you are the man! It's game time. Suit up and give it a go.

Here's the deal. I'll share ideas on some practical things to do. Simply, what we did to get through this crap. These include ways to help a partner in need and things to keep you sane while doing it (no guarantees). Breast cancer is, by all accounts, one hell of a ride. With any luck at all, you'll end up at the bottom of the hill, and all will be well. Otherwise, why would you buy a ticket and give it a shot? Well, LOVE will inspire you to do some pretty crazy things, and in this case, it should drive you to be the real guy. The one someone else leans on for support and looks to for help. You the MAN? Or are you grabbing the remote?

I was going to ask some famous people to include their advice in this manual, but there were two problems with that approach. First, I don't know anyone famous. Second, this is intended to be a primer. Short and to the point. I know from experience that if it's too long or complex you aren't going to read it. **I am not offering medical advice. That you need to get from a specialist who can guide you through health care decisions.** The main intent here is to offer some practical suggestions that were passed on to me or ideas that I just stumbled upon. It's not perfect, but it will give you a jump-start in understanding breast cancer, what to expect, and how to support your partner.

CHAPTER 2

Our Story

Okay, first—our story in brief. It will be different than your experience. Based on what we've heard and read, each breast cancer case is unique. Here's how it went down for us on August 1, 2007.

Ann, my wife of now twenty-five years, was off to Annapolis to meet with her doctor. This was a follow-up to surgery she'd had the week before to remove some cysts from her breasts. She'd had the cysts for about six years. They'd been repeatedly checked and were nothing to worry about. Plus, Ann had mammograms religiously. We were fairly comfortable that all was okey-dokey. Nonetheless, she decided that since she was now retired, she'd have the cysts removed. It was time to quit wondering about them.

So off she goes. We'd relocated to Maryland's eastern shore from a four-year assignment in London the year before, and this full-time togetherness thing was taking its toll. A little alone time met my needs perfectly. Ann's plan was to spend her obligatory ten minutes with the doctor, then squander the rest of the day shopping. Unused to so much free time, Ann was still looking for things to fill her day and shopping was becoming more than a passing fancy. It all seemed to fit.

She called me at 11:00 AM. The world tilted! She asked me to come to Annapolis right away and the tone of her voice kept me from making any of my normal wise-ass comments when I asked why.

She responded, "The surgeon just told me I have breast cancer."

Time stopped! The world went blank. Numbness set in, and I was momentarily speechless.

In my silence, Ann spoke again. "They've arranged for me to see a specialist at the Anne Arundel Breast Center right away. I think you need to be here."

I snapped out of my stupor. "I'm on the way. I'll be there with you as soon as I can. Just hang on, Honey, we'll get through this together."

Annapolis is an hour away, and Ann eventually driving herself home did not seem a viable option. I called buddy and neighbor Ben Battaglino.

"I need to get to Annapolis right now, and I need you to take me," I said.

Ben responded immediately. "Be there in five minutes."

With no questions asked, Ben just dropped everything and came. It's what friends do!

Upon arriving at the Center, I found Ann in consultation with the breast surgeon, a young woman with impressive credentials. Ann and I kissed, held hands, listened, and took notes. She cried, while I tried to be helpful. The doctor was pulled out of the room for a few minutes (by design?), and I made my first blunder.

"Ann, you need to quit crying. It's very unprofessional in front of these people."

Her look would have frozen water. Then she offered a wry hint of a smile and said, "Bob, you are such a jerk!"

I took my licking like a man and totally agreed. In my defense, I think I just wanted her to stay engaged to what they were saying. It was going to take both of us to understand what was going on, and I felt ill-equipped to do it by myself. Hell, I was scared to death. Lord knows Ann was. At this point, the doctor might as well have been speaking in tongues for as little as I understood.

The breast surgeon returned and explained what had happened. None of the original cysts were the problem, but upon their removal, our original surgeon had seen some odd-looking tissue and excised it. He had mentioned this to Ann following surgery but said he felt certain it was nothing to worry about. However, after testing the tissue, it turned out to be a 3.2 cm tumor and the margins weren't clean—meaning he didn't get it all. The bottom line, as now explained by the breast surgeon, was that Ann had invasive lobular carcinoma of the left breast.

As a result, the breast surgeon didn't feel a lumpectomy was appropriate because she couldn't be certain where to go in and get the remaining tumor. She recommended a mastectomy of the left breast, which would likely be followed by chemotherapy. The options around reconstruction were also introduced. To top it off, the timeline discussed from this point to the completion of breast reconstruction was almost a year. What a shock. It was like being in a whirlwind. So many things were coming at once when we hadn't even gotten our heads around the idea that cancer had entered our life.

I was dumbfounded to find out that one in every eight American women gets breast cancer. How could that be? Plus, lobular cancer accounts for only 10-15 percent of breast cancers, and it is not easily detectable. It grows more like tentacles, versus a lump that is more easily detected by feel and in mammograms. Bottom line, we were just lucky, and thankful, that the cancer was found. Up to this point, Ann and her family felt they were pretty safe. Her maternal grandmother had breast cancer at age forty-four. When brain cancer occurred eighteen years later, she died. Ann's grandmother had two daughters and one son. They collectively had eleven granddaughters. None, until Ann, had developed breast cancer, so the family's response to the one-in-eight ratio was low. The clan had erroneously thought they had beaten the odds.

What next after getting the bad news? Here's what I suggest. Guys, start taking notes and grabbing brochures (more of this under "Getting Organized"). Be supportive, loving, caring, and grab her hand. Stay close! Start using "we."

"We will get thru this."

"We will beat this."

"We will, we will, we will."

Apparently, I use "we" a lot. I guess you can overdo it, but it *is* a journey together. One of my more clever overuses of "we" occurred some weeks later as Ann was rolled on the gurney from the Preop Area to the Operating Room for her mastectomy.

"Be tough, kid," I said. "We're going to get through this."

Ann's response still rings in my ears. "What is this 'we' shit, Tonto?" Her retort resulted in a number of grins around the room.

The best thing you can do early on in this process is to be patient. Don't rush to judge what course of treatment is best. Put a clamp on your need to kill the problem and make a decision. Help your partner realize that there will be a lot of tests like an EKG, mammogram, ultrasound, and blood work. And, if you're smart, there will be physician consultations for second and third opinions thrown in for good measure. Never make a choice before you have to. Do not be pushed by anyone, and I mean *anyone*, to make a decision before you are both comfortable with the selected course of action.

CHAPTER 3

Managing the Process

You will find out about cancer in many different ways. No matter how you find out, it will be a shock beyond your ken. Nothing prepares you for how to handle this! So, where do you start? Some strong advice: PROCESS is the key word.

I don't know for sure, but you will likely go through all the traditional emotions—denial, why me, it's not true, etc. Fine! Grab on to all that B.S. and let it roll. You have twenty-four to forty-eight hours. Let the tears rain, the emotions soar, and go with the flow. After a day or two, suck it up and get hold of the situation. Easy to say? Of course! Easy to do? No!

Come to grips with the fact that you both are either into a process that you can manage or a process that can manage you. Ann and I are strong proponents of managing the process. There are two primary reasons for this.

First, you have just been told an ugly truth about which you apparently have no control. You did not deserve this, and you are feeling helpless. If you decide to manage the process then you are back in the driver's seat. You decide which doctors to see, where to seek treatment and what treatment seems best for you. You have the ability to research information, talk to experts, friends, family, other cancer survivors, use the Internet, read, and get up-to-speed on the lingo and medical terms that will be thrown at you. If you spend too much time feeling sorry for yourself and being a victim, you will quickly be behind the power curve.

You may say, "Well what's the point? They are going to tell us what to do anyway!" The problem with that approach is that treating breast cancer is not a black and white situation. The two of you will have choices to make around a lumpectomy versus mastectomy (or not), reconstruction, radiation, chemotherapy, and on it goes. Informed decisions are always better than just following someone's suggestion. This is the case with any serious illness. **Keep in mind that there is only one acceptable end-game and that is to live and beat this disease.**

This needs to be a shared responsibility. One of you may take the lead on this, but you both need to be engaged. No one person can reasonably expect to assimilate all the information that will come your way and make a good decision. Guys, you need to pony-up and dig in. Start and end the process with a "no regrets" mindset, so when you look back on the experience you will know you did all you could.

Second, you need to manage this process because you'll get diverse information from surgeons, nurses, oncologists, etc. There is nothing sinister or intentionally misleading going on. It's like different shades of the same color. This is particularly disturbing to rat killers who think "I've got a problem, so I've got to nuke it." This process is like going through a maze...so many decisions and options. The protocols for treatment are constantly changing, all designed to improve your odds for reaching the end-game. Don't get overwhelmed or frustrated. If you do, back-off. Review what you know, which decisions you have already reached, and think about what needs to come next. What I've found helpful is to use a "helicopter approach." Every once in a while, lift off and look at the big picture. This may allow you to put the details into perspective and stop scratching your head.

When we first learned about Ann's cancer, our immediate reaction was to fly to Houston for a second opinion at M.D. Anderson Cancer Center. It is considered one of the best cancer treatment facilities in the world. Having lived in Houston for most of our careers, this seemed like an obvious choice, and one with which we would be comfortable. After all, we had only lived in Maryland about a year. In fact, we strongly considered having surgery and everything else in

Texas. Then we stepped back from the panic and looked at the big picture. This alternative would require frequent trips from Maryland to Texas and a place to stay while there. Ann and I love the comforts of our home, and the idea of getting on an airplane when she wasn't feeling good caused us to reconsider. So, we decided not to even go for the second opinion in Houston and focused our treatment options in Maryland and Washington D.C. We chose Johns Hopkins Hospital in Baltimore, an easy two-hour drive away. The helicopter view saved us on this one!

This whole concept of getting different information from different doctors is just so foreign to some of us that it's mind-boggling. On some intellectual level, I suppose we can resonate. But, when you grew up thinking these all-knowing, god-like individuals could cure you from any malady, to even think about questioning them was crazy. Well guess what? You need to get over that pretty quick. It's imperative that you question everything and everybody constantly. You are managing this process. You are the decision maker. You can't help your partner make the right decision unless you are knowledgeable about the choices.

Know what else? All doctors are not created equal. They may not have the same experience or be on the leading edge of technology. You may love your local GP—hell if you're lucky, they may even speak English well. But, if you've got the "Big C" in your life, you want the "A-team," with a breast cancer pro at your side. If you can get your arms around the fact that some doctors are better than others, then you can see why you had better manage this process, because you will have to help choose the best path.

This is a very important area where you can contribute. You need to help your mate weigh the pros and cons around options and what is best for her. The proverbial, "Whatever you think dear!" ain't gonna work. This has got to be a team effort!

And avoid the "what if" thing. This is particularly hard to do. What if they say this or the test shows this or that? What comes to mind is the sports analogy of playing one game at a time. Well, in this case, it's one decision at a time. Don't get ahead of yourself. If you do, it can be overwhelming. If you follow one step at a time, one decision at a time, you'll be better able to manage the situation.

Remember...MANAGE THE PROCESS.

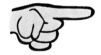 **PARTNER TIPS**

This is an ongoing process with lots of decisions and information to be managed. Listed below are tips regarding a few areas that require almost immediate attention.

Second/Third Opinions —Take the time to get a second and/or third opinion about the best course of action. Don't be shy in telling the first doctor you speak with that you want a second opinion. We even asked the first surgical oncologist for her input on other doctors to talk to and she gave us three names. We went to one of those for a second opinion. In the end, we didn't make our decision just on what the chosen doctor recommended and his qualifications. We also considered our fit with the style of each physician and what we'd be most comfortable with. While he wouldn't be a fit for everyone, we chose the in-your-face, tell-it-like-it-is doctor, who turned out to be perfect for us.

The "A-Team"—You're likely looking at a whole team of doctors—possibly a breast surgeon (who cuts out the cancer), a radiation oncologist (physician who treats cancer patients with radiation therapy), a medical oncologist (physician who treats cancer with chemo and other drugs—often referred to as your oncologist) and a plastic/reconstruction surgeon. Get the best team of doctors and hospital you can, but balance this decision with other factors like need, location, etc. For example, one of the doctors noted that lobular breast cancer is more rare than ductal. However, in his words, we were still "dealing with a horse, not a zebra." He said that if Ann had a zebra (rare) cancer, then we should go to the best doctor and hospital in the world for that cancer. But, with breast cancer being so common, many large cities have highly rated breast cancer doctors, hospitals, and treatment centers.

Think about what works best for each stage of the process. The doctors don't all have to come from the same institution. You want a surgical oncologist and plastic surgeon that work with breast cancer on a regular basis, so you may need to drive further for that. Getting chemo and radiation is tough enough without adding a long drive to the equation, so having your medical oncologist and/or radiation oncologist close by is useful. Additionally, the medical oncologist often becomes the go-to doctor for much of the ongoing cancer care, so easy access is a plus.

CHAPTER 4

Our Plan of Attack and Timeline

So how does one understand that which is unfathomable or subject to the frailties of man? I'm not really sure, but the helicopter approach will benefit you in this area. Think of major milestones...big pieces that are accomplished so you can move on to the next hurdle. It's the only way to go, lest you become totally overwhelmed and frustrated with the pace of progress.

We've included our timeline and plan of attack below, which may help in understanding what to expect medically. At the end of the book, you'll find the overall treatment timeline with tips on how to support your loved one in each stage. All in all, the duration of Ann's recovery was about eighteen months from the time of diagnosis until we got into a run-and-maintain mode. That is not to say that life stopped during this period. See the following example.

In May 2008, we decided to take a vacation. Ann was postchemo, and this was her first big adventure out since her cancer diagnosis nine months earlier. We met friends Jo and Tim in Yellowstone National Park and stayed at the Old Faithful Inn, right next to the geyser. After breakfast, we decided to meet in forty-five minutes and start our day's expedition searching for animals. Tim went to the car to putz with his camera, and Jo went shopping. I enjoyed some solitude with a newspaper, while Annie moseyed around looking for the post office. This effort was complicated by her directional disorder known as The-Sun-Comes-Up-In-The-West, and where sometimes north could be south. About five minutes later, Ann met Mr. Grizzly

Bear, who was only about a hundred yards away. He probably thought Annie, dressed in her white quilted jacket, was the biggest rabbit in the world. The race was on! I'm happy to say Ann won, due to a generous head start. Tim actually got pictures as the bear left Ann and raced through the parking lot, oblivious to all the people screaming and jumping into any car available. I exited the hotel to a lot of honking horns and a wife that was yelling, "There's a bear…a REALLY BIG BEAR, and it just chased me!" With my normal approach to situations like this, I told Ann to get a grip on reality. Wrong move once again. After debriefing, it was apparent that Annie was back in the game big-time. See a bear, run from the bear (not the preferred approach), and don't have a heart attack. I was a really happy camper!

I digress. The major point here is that it was not eighteen months of lying around the house. There were plenty of ups and downs. Because every breast cancer case is unique, the plan of attack and time needed to kill the problem is specific to each individual. This involves getting input from others, including your surgeons and oncologist. Putting it all together to understand the general flow of events, the associated timeline, and what to expect will help you both cope with the future. Two things to remember in doing this: 1) whatever you start with is not what it ultimately will be, and 2) remain flexible. Never forget the end-game; you are on a journey with only one acceptable outcome. A bit arduous, but given a little patience, it's doable.

Our Treatment Timeline

Diagnosis & Plan of Attack	Surgery & Treatment	Recuperation & Reconstruction	Follow Up
About 1 1/2–2 Months.	About 6–7 Months	About 7–9 Months	Ongoing
2007	**2007**	**2008**	**2009**
8/1—Told had breast cancer	9/20—Mastectomy	3/1 to 6/30—Body recuperates from chemo	Continue daily hormone therapy pills for five years
8/8—Second opinion at Johns Hopkins	9/26—Remove drain	4/16 to 5/8—Four expander inflations	Periodic check-ups: blood tests, MRIs, bone density scans, mammograms, etc.
8/2 to 9/19	10/8 to 10/23—Three expander inflations	6/19—Surgery to remove expander & insert implant	
—More tests	10/23 to 12/4—Biweekly chemo treatments (Adriamycin & Cytoxan) with Neulasta injection following each to boost white blood cells	9/18—Reconstruct nipple	
—Doctor consultations			
—Sort insurance coverage		12/12—Redo of nipple reconstruction	
— Tell family & friends			
	11/7—Hair falling out		
	11/9—Shaved head	**2009**	
		1/15—Areola tattoo	
	12/5/07 to 1/1/08—Break between chemo drugs		
	2008		
	1/2 to 3/4—Tri-weekly chemo treatments (Taxotere)		
	1/08—Eyelashes & brows fall out		
	4/3—Start daily hormone therapy pills (Femara)		

CHAPTER 5

Telling Others

"I don't want anyone to know...why me...I'll be disfig-ured...what will people think...I'm sick and I'm going to my room...I'm just going to deal with this on my own...it is what it is...I don't want the looks from others...no one needs to know!"

I'm pretty sure we went through most of these responses. Who, if anyone, should you tell that you have breast cancer (BC)? When and how much do you tell them? These are very difficult decisions to make. I daresay, as a caretaker, you may have an opinion on these choices that is different from your partner's. You may be in some kind of denial yourself or in a funky I-don't-want-things-to-change state. Being overprotective, you just may not believe what is happening. Whatever the feelings, I would urge you to get them under control. You can influence the decision to tell others and probably should, given the decision should be a joint one. Ultimately, it will be your partner who carries the day. How she chooses to deal with telling others will depend on her style, relationship with family and friends, and her BC situation. Women are incredible creatures who will go to great lengths to protect the ones they love and maintain the air of nor-malcy if it means that the unit (family) will remain whole and func-tioning properly. I don't know where this comes from...maybe it's genetic or just conditioning, but I've seen it too often to ignore it. So, agree on a communications plan that best fits your overall needs.

I understand a woman going stealth because she doesn't want to show any weakness in a male-dominated work environment. Also, some women don't want to share their personal situations because they like to keep their private life to themselves. But let's get real! There are few secrets, especially in business, the neighborhood, or among family and friends. I don't know how it happens, but the word always…ALWAYS…leaks out sooner or later. So, if you choose to be silent, keep in mind the only one you may be fooling is yourself.

My personal bias is to tell others when it seems appropriate—in your own way, on your own timeline, and with the appropriate amount of information. They're going to find out eventually anyway, so why not manage this process yourselves? It strikes me that there may be three camps around how to do this.

First, is the "Let Me Tell the World" approach. Announce early, often and loud! Second, is the ultra-private tactic of "No One Needs to Know." It's personal and nobody else's business. The third option is what we did after debating it for almost a week. We told people when we were ready and had a bit more data on Ann's diagnosis. The trick on this one is to have sufficient information to answer the plethora of questions that come at you, versus waiting too long, whereby the ones you love feel left out. Whatever works, works! But it should be a considered decision by both of you.

As for us, we told immediate family first and then moved to extended family and closest friends. At some point we got to "who cares who knows" and sent out an e-mail to many others so no one would be left out of the news. It's pretty damn obvious that something is going on when your hair starts coming out. Personally, I think trying to go stealth on this is wrong. You will lose out on the support of others who have been there, beaten the big C down, and can help your partner understand what's going on. But, again this is a very personal decision and one with which you both need to be comfortable.

Telling children is obviously a unique subset of the above. Our children are grown, so we did not face the same challenge as those of you with children still living at home, but granddaughters Kari and Kylie required careful planning. Here is some advice we've received from others: tell the children as soon as possible. Don't attempt to keep it a secret, as they will quickly sense a problem brewing and begin to imagine all sorts of possibilities. Keep the discussion age-appropriate. Young children need simple reassuring words, but older kids expect, and can handle, more information. Pictures may work for small children to explain where mom is sick. Playing with wigs and bandanas may help prepare them for the inevitable changes in appearance. It's okay to use the word "cancer" in the discussion, as they are going to hear others talking about it and need to be familiar with the term. So, be honest but don't over do it with more information than they need to know. Let them ask questions and keep the conversation going over time. As soon as you start telling a larger circle of friends and family, make sure to include some people that can support your children (like teachers, parents of their friends, etc.).

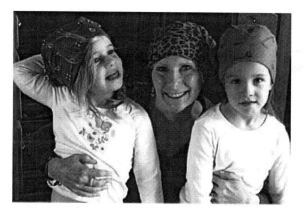

Kylie and Kari learn about baldness and have fun with bandanas.

Lastly, I hate to state the obvious, but the fewer people that know, the less support you will have. Support is a very KEY ingredient. This is not regarding you per se but about your loved one. She needs all she can get. This is not to say that you don't give enough or care enough. It's just that she needs all that's available. MAKE IT HAPPEN!

CHAPTER 6

Breast Cancer 101

"You have invasive lobular breast cancer— a 3.2 cm tumor — inked margins positive."

The words we heard from the breast surgeon were like blinking red lights. They didn't sound good, but what did they really mean? Panic began to set in!

I assume that if you are reading this primer, then you have already been initiated to the Land of Breast Cancer, as we were. Breast cancer terminology includes many strange and fancy words that can be hard to take in, understand, and remember—even after multiple explanations.

A key piece of information for us was learning that breast cancers are as varied as the women affected by them. By looking at the many different characteristics of the cancer, your doctor can size up the cancer's "personality." For example, is the tumor small and low-key? Is it angry, aggressive, and fast-moving? Or is it very large but easy-going? Is its behavior wild and unpredictable, or does it play by the rules? Many tests and analyses will be done to figure out the unique traits of the cancer. These test results will give you and your doctor answers to important questions.

The list of terms below doesn't come close to covering everything, but it is vocabulary that you should basically understand. My advice? Recognize that this is like a puzzle. You will keep getting new information that adds to the overall diagnosis and helps you and your partner determine the appropriate course of action. Read a lot.

Heaven knows, you will be given lots of brochures and books to consume.

Remember, the smartest patients are often the worst patients. Push, nudge, and ask questions. I can't reinforce it enough—you must manage the process!

Now, since I have already hinted as to the kind of man I am, I can also add that I am not that into details. I generally like the big picture. So what follows was written by Ann. She is detail-oriented but readily admits she doesn't do humor. Hence, we both apologize for the lack of wit in the following information, but it doesn't really lend itself to that anyway. Ann gathered this data from the pile of books she'd been given and numerous Web sites on BC. **But remember that we are not doctors and new facts are constantly evolving. This is just a starter to use as a quick reference. You will need to dig into the details of your partner's diagnosis together with your doctors.**

Breast Cancer Basics

Types of Breast Cancer—The two most common types of breast cancer are ***ductal and lobular.*** Ductal involves the ducts, or tiny tubes in the breast, through which milk flows to the nipple. Lobular cancer involves the lobules which are the milk-making glands at the end of the ducts. Other types of breast cancer are less common and include colloid, medullary, tubular, inflammatory, and adenocystic.

Non-invasive ("in situ") or Invasive—The single most important factor in the personality of any breast cancer is whether it is non-invasive or invasive.

Non-invasive, also called in situ, refers to tumors that have not grown beyond their original place of origin, the ducts or lobules.

- *Ductal Carcinoma in situ (DCIS)*—ductal cancer cells that have not grown outside the ducts. DCIS is sometimes called a pre-cancer and usually cannot be felt as a lump. Hence, women are encouraged to have annual mammograms to help find it at an early stage.

- *Lobular Carcinoma in situ (LCIS)*—lobular cells that are not normal and have not grown outside the lobules. LCIS is generally not considered a true breast cancer, as is DCIS.

Invasive cancer, also called infiltrating, has spread outside the duct or lobules into normal tissue inside the breast. Invasive cancers are much more serious than non-invasive, and can spread to other parts of the body through the bloodstream and lymphatic system.

- *Invasive Ductal Carcinoma (IDC)*—a cancer that begins in the milk duct but grows into the normal breast tissue around it. About 70-80 percent of all breast cancers are invasive ductal carcinoma.

- *Invasive Lobular Carcinoma (ILC)*—a cancer that starts inside the milk-making gland but grows into the normal breast tissue around it. It accounts for about 10 to 15 percent of invasive breast cancers.

Margins—When cancer cells are excised from the breast, the surgeon tries to remove the whole cancer with an extra area or "margin" of normal tissue around it. This is to be sure that all of the cancer is removed. The tissue around the very edge of what was removed is microscopically examined to see if it is free of cancer cells. The pathologist also measures the distance between the cancer cells and the outer edge of the tissue.

Margins around a cancer are described in three ways:

- Negative—No cancer cells can be seen at the outer edge. Usually, no more surgery is needed.

- Positive—Cancer cells come right out to the edge of the tissue. More surgery may be needed.

- Close—Cancer cells are close to the edge of the tissue but not right at the edge. More surgery may be needed.

Spread—Your doctors will also try to determine if the cancer has spread. The spread of breast cancer is usually referred to in the following ways: 1) Local—means the cancer is confined within the breast, 2) Regional—means the lymph nodes, primarily those in the armpit, are involved, and 3) Distant—means the cancer is also present in other parts of the body.

Size—Tumors are measured in centimeters (cm). Size matters when it comes to breast cancer, but size is only one of the personality features to be considered. Keep in mind that the cancer can be small but bullish or large and mild-mannered.

Lymph Node Involvement—The breast has a network of blood vessels and lymph channels that connect breast tissue to other parts of the body. These are like highways that carry fluid and blood around the body, bringing in nourishment and removing the waste products of cell life. They connect the breast tissue to other parts of the body. Lymph fluid leaves the breast and goes back to the bloodstream. Lymph nodes are filters along the lymph fluid channels that try to catch cancer cells so that they don't spread elsewhere. Knowing whether you have cancer cells in the nodes is a critical piece of information about the risk of the cancer spreading. If the nodes have some cancer cells in them they are called positive. Where no invasion is found, the nodes are negative. In most cases, the more extensive the lymph node involvement, the more aggressive the cancer is. But the extent of disease within a particular lymph node is less important than the total number of lymph nodes affected. The more lymph nodes that are involved, the more threatening the cancer may be.

Sentinel Node Biopsy—Your doctor may want to do a biopsy of a key lymph node called the sentinel node. The sentinel node is the first in line as fluid drains from the breast and the node most likely to contain escaped cancer cells. During the procedure, a radioactive substance and/or blue dye is injected into the area around the tumor. Lymphatic vessels carry these materials to the sentinel node. After identifying the node, the doctor removes it to determine if it is cancer free. If cancer is found, surgery is generally performed to remove more of the lymph nodes for further testing.

Stages of Breast Cancer—Many doctors categorize a cancer according to an established breast cancer staging system based on: 1) the size of the tumor measured in centimeters with 1cm equaling .39 inches, 2) the extent to which the tumor is involved with the skin, muscles, and other tissues next to it, and 3) lymph node involvement. The purpose of the staging system is to help organize some of the cancer's different factors and personality features into categories in order to facilitate treatment decisions and formulate a prognosis. Clinical studies of breast cancer treatments are partly organized by the staging system, so knowing your stage is another important piece of information. Below are high level descriptions, as they can be much more specific with subcategories within a stage (e.g., multiple subcategories at Stage II and III).

Stage 0	Describes non-invasive or in situ breast cancer. DCIS cancer cells remain in the duct, and LCIS cells stay in the lobules.
Stage I	Describes invasive breast cancer. Cancer cells break through or invade the neighboring normal tissue. The tumor is less than 2 cm, and no lymph nodes are involved.
Stage II	Cancer has spread from the ducts or lobules into the surrounding breast tissue. The tumor is 2-5 cm. Sometimes there is lymph node involvement.
Stage III	Tumors may be larger than 5 cm and the cancer may or may not have spread to nodes. Or, in some cases, the tumor is smaller with several nodes involved. A concern at Stage III is that the tumor

spreads to other local areas, such as the breast skin, chest wall, or internal mammary lymph nodes.

Stage IV   Commonly known as metastatic breast cancer. The cancer has spread to other parts of the body, such as the brain, lung, bones or liver.

STOP! Take a break. Go get a cup of coffee or other beverage of your choice. Take a short walk. Reflect on what you've read so far, as this can be a bit overwhelming. Then come back and skim what you've already read in this section. Highlight relevant information and make notes on your own situation. Then, read on.

Grade—Grade compares cancer cells to normal breast cells. It relates to cell growth and how much the tumor cells look like cancer. Poorly differentiated cells may predict a more aggressive cancer, but not necessarily so. In fact, most breast cancers are either moderately or poorly differentiated, so don't jump to conclusions on what this ultimately means.

Grade 1   Cancer cells still look a lot like normal cells. They might be referred to as "well-differentiated" and are usually slow growing.

Grade 2   Cancer cells do not look like normal cells and may be called "moderately differentiated." These cells have either an average or fast growth rate and tend to stick together.

Grade 3   Cancer cells are wilder looking or poorly differentiated. They tend to be fast growing, disorganized,
irregularly shaped, and stick together.

Rate of growth—The proportion of cancer cells dividing and making new cells varies from tumor to tumor. This helps to predict how
aggressive a cancer is, with the thought being that the more they
divide, the more aggressive they are. Your doctor may order a special
test, called *S-phase fraction or Ki-67*, to determine if the cells are
growing at a faster than normal rate. Because results from these
screenings can be iffy, doctors use them as indicators but rely more
on other characteristics and tests.

Ploidy—Do the cancer cells have a normal number of chromosomes? Doctors also use ploidy, a measurement of the number of
chromosomes present in cancer cells, to determine how fast a tumor
may be growing. *Diploid* cancer cells have a normal number of chromosomes. *Aneuploid* cells have more chromosomes than normal
because they are growing faster than normal. Ploidy is just one factor in the grand scheme of a cancer's personality, but we were told
this feature, on its own, does not have a major impact on your outcome, as 70 percent of breast cancer tumors are aneuploid.

HER-2—Does the cancer have genes that are normal? HER-2, also
called HER-2/neu, is a gene that produces a type of receptor (HER-
2 receptor) that helps cancer cells grow. About one out of four breast
cancers has too many copies of this gene, generally resulting in a
faster growing cancer. However, these cancers do respond well to
HER-2 anti-antibody therapy. There are two tests for HER-2:

- *IHC test* (IHC stands for immunohistochemistry)—The IHC
  test shows if there is too much HER-2 receptor protein in the
  cancer cells. The results of the IHC test can be 0 (negative),
  1+ (negative), 2+ (borderline), or 3+ (positive).

- *FISH test* (FISH stands for fluorescence in situ hybridiza-
  tion)—The FISH test shows if there are too many copies of
  the HER-2 gene in the cancer cells. The results of the FISH
  test can be "positive" (extra copies) or "negative" (normal
  number of copies).

Due to cost and the difficulty of the FISH test, screening is often done with the IHC test first. If the result of it is 2+, make sure you get a FISH test. Cancers that test IHC 3+ or FISH "positive" will respond best to therapy that works against HER-2.

Hormone Receptors—Hormone receptors are like ears on breast cells that listen to signals from hormones. These signals "turn on" growth in breast cells that have receptors. A tumor is called *"ER-positive"* if it has receptors for the hormone estrogen. It is called *"PR-positive"* if it has receptors for the hormone progesterone. Breast cells that do not have receptors are "negative" for these hormones. Breast cancers that are ER-positive or PR-positive, or both, tend to respond well to hormone therapy. These cancers can be treated with medicine that reduces the estrogen in your body. They can also be treated with medicine that keeps estrogen away from the receptors. If the cancer has no hormone receptors, there are still very effective treatments available. Results of the hormone receptor test are written in one of these three ways:

1) The percent of cells that have receptors out of one hundred cells tested. You will see a number between 0 percent (no receptors) and 100 percent (all have receptors).
2) A number between zero and three. This translates as: 0 (no receptors), 1+ (a small number), 2+ (a medium number), or 3+ (a large number of receptors).
3) You will also see the word "positive" or "negative."

Hormone Therapy—This is cancer treatment using pills that remove, block, or add hormones to the body Your oncologist will discuss the potential benefits of the medication. It is taken for five years and reduces the odds of cancer reoccurring. Typical names include tamoxifen, anastrazole (Arimidex) and letrozole (Femara).

Chemotherapy—Chemo is given using very powerful drugs intended to destroy cancer cells or make them less active. It treats the entire body and, as such, is known as a systemic treatment. Typical drugs include Adriamycin, Cytoxan, Taxol and Taxotere. They are administered at set one- to three-week intervals determined by your oncologist.

Radiation Therapy—Women who undergo a lumpectomy generally receive radiation afterwards. Unlike chemo, radiation is a local treatment, meaning it affects only the part of the body that is radiated. It bombards the breast, chest wall, and/or armpit with X-rays to damage and destroy cancer cells. Treatments are daily, usually Monday through Friday, for five to seven weeks.

* * *

After numerous tests, both pre- and postsurgery, this is what the pieces of the puzzle told us. Ann was in Stage IIB because her left breast tumor was 3.2 cm with positive lymph nodes. The cancer had spread to one of the six lymph nodes removed, so the cancer could also have spread outside the breast. As is common, the many tests conducted didn't all point to the same conclusion, with results being somewhat mixed on growth rate and aggressiveness. The tumor showed a low-to-intermediate grade, meaning the cancer cells looked somewhat, but not totally, normal. The IHC and FISH tests were favorable in that she didn't have too many of the HER-2 genes and receptors that predict faster growth. However, the Ki-67 test indicated a slightly faster-than-normal growth rate. And, as with the majority of breast cancers, aneuploid cells were found. Tests on the breast tissue removed during the mastectomy revealed there had also been extensive residual lobular carcinoma in situ. The breast surgeon and the oncologist both described Ann's cancer as somewhat in the middle of good and bad—it wasn't a friendly cancer but could be much worse. We felt relieved.

Because there was lymph node involvement, the chemotherapy would use three versus two drugs and be extended from four treatments to eight. Ann wouldn't need radiation since it is targeted to decreasing the recurrence of cancer within the breast, which had now been removed. Ann had tested ER/PR positive so hormonal therapy was recommended. This therapy (pills) would start after chemo and continue for five years to further reduce the risk of recurrence. The oncologist said the risk of the cancer recurring in the next ten years was about 35 percent, but with both the chemo and hormone therapy, the risk could be reduced to 15 percent. The hormone therapy would also reduce the risk of cancer occurring in the healthy right breast.

Stop again. As noted, we are not medical practitioners. Also, since this information continues to change, updated data may be required to fully prepare for conversations with your doctor.

Now take a long breath and then reread this section. Summarize what you know about your partner's diagnosis and what questions you have. Don't feel stupid that you may need to ask your doctor about issues that were previously discussed. I certainly did. This is complicated; little ends up as straightforward as you'd like.

Take a breath or two. Relax.

CHAPTER 7

Get Organized and Pissed Off

Now, you may be wondering how these thoughts—getting organized and pissed off—actually mix. Well, you've got to have a bunch of attitude as you go through this. You need an edge to you that shows you are managing the process, and you're in charge. You'll make the decisions, but only after you have all the data and time to reflect. You won't be pushed into anything you don't understand, and you won't be herded. For myself, I had to be a bit pissed off to get that edge. And I was. Life had been going along pretty well and then this happened. So, I didn't have to work too hard at getting an edge.

Plus, you'll need it to get organized. Who wants to be all that organized when you're retired, as I was? Who needs it? Well, this is one of those things that requires a lot of organization.

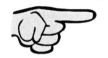 **PARTNER TIPS**

The best bet is to get a big binder and start filling it up with information. Subject matters go like this:

Contacts—Keep tabs and phone numbers/addresses/etc., of every doctor, nurse, expert, or resource that you talk to. This will get very long— much longer than you can imagine as the tests pile up—but you will reference it frequently. Make sure you are clear on who to contact in the evenings and on weekends, should the need arise.

Chronology—Create one as you go along. Who you talked to, when and what they had to say or recommend. This is an excellent tool when you get confused and can't quite remember what was said. It also allows you to easily compare what everyone is saying to help you formulate questions. Doctor so and so said "x" but the other doctor said "y," so what gives? You will be faced with a few of these as you struggle to make decisions. Use your newfound ATTITUDE, and get in someone's face when you seem to have contradictory input. For example, one doctor recommended that Ann go through sixteen weeks of chemo, and then have the mastectomy. He had no clinical data to support this recommendation but truly thought it was a better protocol. Absent a large tumor you needed to shrink (most of Ann's had already been removed), the logic was not compelling. I confirmed this with another surgeon. We went another route. If you aren't organized and managing all that is going on with an attitude, it's just too easy to go along with the expert who is sitting in front of you.

Copies—Get copies of everything you can. Every test, X-ray, result, diagnosis, everything. There is a very practical reason for this. Everybody wants to see the same stuff. Getting things moved from one doctor or hospital to the next relies on people who are often busy as hell. Guess what? Things get held up, someone forgot, someone didn't get the message. The last thing you want are any more delays than are inherent in the process. Get copies and drag them with you to every appointment. The new doctor wants to see them? Fine. Tell him/her to make a copy from yours.

Actual Records—Mammograms, MRIs, CAT scans, X-rays, etc. Know where they are, as many doctors want to see the real thing. The actual films/CDs for these records get passed around from one doctor to the next. The medical facility will often help with the transport of such records, but whether they are shipped or hand-carried, you need to keep track of where these records land. Again, with everything going on, it's easy to forget where the records are, and you're going to need them on multiple occasions. To the extent possible, get copies of written reports, as well. Get a nice big tote bag to drag all this stuff around with you.

Tests—Keep a separate list of all the tests performed, the date, and who ordered them. This is a helpful reference, as well. Trust me, it all starts to run together, so a written record is immensely helpful.

Notes—This is a bit painful, but both of you need to take notes at every meeting. By adding these observations together, you will have a better understanding of what actually went down. Keep these records and use them as a reference. This is particularly helpful for developing questions for the next doctor or hospital.

Medical Insurance—If you have insurance, feel blessed. Get working on understanding your coverage. What's your deductible? Do you have one? Do you have an in-network and out-of-network option? Does your coverage offer expert advice counselors? Are second opinions covered? Do you need to be referred to specialists or can you make appointments directly? Are the doctors you are considering covered by your plan? What percent of surgery costs are covered? Will you be reimbursed for a wig, if needed, etc.? Get on top of this. If you don't, it will drive you crazy. Ask yourself if money will drive your decisions. Be honest with yourself, as this is not a cheap trip. Discuss it between the two of you. No hidden agendas allowed.

No Medical Insurance—Many people faced with breast cancer don't have insurance, are underinsured, or have huge deductibles. If you are reading this, you likely already have a preliminary diagnosis and have seen a medical specialist. Get their input regarding resources available. You can also seek advice from your local county health department, nearby breast cancer or cancer centers, and cancer support groups. Network the dickens out of these organizations to understand what options are available.

Medical Bills and Receipts—Organize these and keep them filed separately from everything else. As it turns out, I found bills to be a major annoyance. They will float in totally outside any expected time context. Doctors and hospitals often bill separately. And, labs are truly alien entities. Tracking our bills is something we should have started sooner. You may well be able to go online to your medical provider's Web site to check the status of bills paid, but nothing beats some old fashioned record keeping. Be warned! Organize this or pull your hair out.

Questions—Keep a running list of the questions you had and the responses received. Again, this is helpful in reviewing where you are and the next step or decision.

If all this doesn't give you attitude, then heaven help you…no, I want to shake your hand, for you are a far better person than I, Gunga Din.

The side benefit to being organized is that it gives you something to do that you that you can control. You can't dictate what people tell you, but you can direct how you use this information and when.

CHAPTER 8

Think Pink

Ann would say that partners of breast cancer patients need to "get in touch with their feminine side." Well, that's great advice, but most of us don't have a clue as to where it is. So what do we do?

It's clearly too late to start thinking like a woman, and wouldn't that just create a world of chaos if we could? However, during this period it will be helpful to understand that men and women often process information differently, communicate differently, and make decisions differently…just to name a few disparities. Face it, we grew up learning a lot of rules, consciously and unconsciously, about being a boy or girl. For example, boys shouldn't cry but girls can. Your partner is going to be very vulnerable during this process, and these differences can get in the way unless you start to "think pink."

In Ann's professional life she was the Global Director of Diversity for a large multi-national corporation. So, I've had more than my fair share of education on this subject. Over the years we've had many opportunities to see these gender differences play out and can even laugh at most of them now.

The classic one for me was when Ann described some problem she had encountered. I listened (usually) and then proceeded to tell her how to solve it. Then she looked at me like I had a turnip sprouting out of my forehead. Our conversations went something like this:

"What?" I ask.

Ann responds. "I just wanted to talk."

"If you didn't want a solution then why did you bring it up?"

"Because I just wanted to talk about it."

I forge ahead, undaunted. "But it's a problem."

"I know."

"Okay, so here's what you do…"

Now I had two turnips sprouting. If I had not shut up, there would have been a whole patch, and she would have dug them all up with a shovel.

When you find yourself in one of these situations (they are in abundance as you try to make decisions) try to be sensitive. At least ask if she's looking for input or just airing out the blankets.

I can't imagine how decisions evolve by you and yours, but this cancer thing will really test you. Ann is very inquisitive and asks a lot of questions, even if they make her look stupid or naïve (in my judgment, of course). On the other hand, I have never needed a lot of data to form an opinion or to make a decision. This is another example of typical gender differences. My process is much more efficient than hers, but the results are a bit iffy from time to time. Anyway, if you are at all like me, you need to curb it, put it in neutral, and try a different approach. Your partner certainly stands no chance of altering her behavior during one of the most stressful times of her life, so the burden is on you. Think pink. Ask open-ended questions…these are the ones without your judgment dripping from every word. Also, just shutting up works well. You want to be helpful? Then go with the flow!

Thinking pink also means to show love and affection like when you were dating, maybe even more. You need to think about this. She is going to endure a truly horrific ordeal. If she has an operation like Ann, she's going to feel disfigured and scarred. Then, when she gets her head around recuperating from that, along comes the chemo, hair loss and a whole host of other physical drawbacks. This goes on for months, and it's no easy road.

This is where you can really be a big help. Hold hands, give her a kiss, tell her you love her, pat her bum, or touch her shoulder. Do any of the many things that show your love and devotion and do them often. There's no time off on this one. These are important moments of truth—your big chance to lay it all on the line. This is what life partners do.

CHAPTER 9

Getting Support

Well, bah humbug! Who needs support anyway? I was convinced I'd provide everything that Ann needed and then some. Every person we met kept bringing this idea up, and I kept mentally blowing them off. I was pretty sure that only the weak and those without attitude would require this support. And from strangers…no way!

Sometimes my ignorance knows no bounds. Obviously, my arrogance has no restraint either. So here I am like a born-again Christian telling you that support makes all the difference. It worked miracles for Ann and me. To know that you are loved, that you are not alone in your struggle, and that those who have traveled this road successfully are standing by your side—is just incredible.

I'm not sure where you will find this support, but it's out there waiting for you. Many people look to their faith for aid. There are all sorts of breast cancer and cancer support groups created for this single purpose. Another source of support is from friends and family who have previously made the breast cancer journey. Heck, there are even support groups just for men. One thing is sure, you will both need support. And for crying out loud, if you need help, please have the courage to ask for it. If offered, accept it. Open yourself up to the magic of loving, caring people. It's a memorable trip.

Our support started almost immediately, as word spread about Ann's diagnosis. The phone started ringing and soon after, cards and flowers arrived. When Ann actually had her mastectomy, things got out of hand. Plants, flowers, balloons, and cards were in abundance.

Our house looked like a funeral home on steroids. I went nuts trying not to kill everything I touched. (Hint: First you water it every few days, or if they are cut flowers, change the water out. If this doesn't work, throw them out when she's not looking and move things around a bit. Most guys are not built for this.)

Rhory and Rhiain, our daughters, called and visited often. They took over Thanksgiving and Christmas dinners at our house, as we weren't traveling much. They even did a lot of the Christmas shopping and wrapping for us, which was a huge stress buster. They made our lives easier, as did our son-in-laws, Doug and Alan. For a couple of beers, they would take on any task around the house or yard.

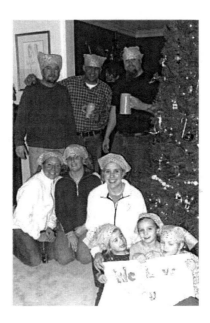

Family Support—pink bandanas rock! (back to front and left to right) Doug, Alan, Jerry, Rhiain, Joelle, Rhory, Kylie, Kari, and Devon.

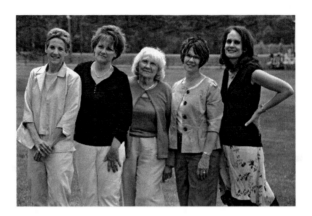

The Indiana Clan —Amy, Karen, Mom (The Sarge), Janis, and Ellen.

Ann's mom, her four sisters, and my brother burnt up the telephone lines. Each of her sisters—Janis, Karen, Amy and Ellen—came from Indiana to personally ensure I was taking care of Ann to their mom's satisfaction. The fact that I call Ann's mother "The Sarge" says something about her expectations, so it was a miracle that I managed to pass the test each time. Brother Doug, who is a professional masseuse, among other things, drove up multiple times from Virginia to give both Ann and me a massage. What a treat that was!

My sister Judy was often on the phone, as were close friends from Texas, The Netherlands and the UK. Our close friend Peggy and her ninety-three-year-old mother Aimee came from New Orleans to cheer us on. We received so many surprises in the mail that the local FedEx and UPS couriers even asked how Ann was doing. One really neat item Ann received was a box sent by the Schlieps from Texas, with gifts for Ann to open before each chemo treatment. What a clever idea! It gave her something to look forward to each time.

Then, there were Ann's designated coaches—friends she asked to help in specific ways. Josie in Houston had breast cancer eleven years earlier, so she became Ann's designated "Cancer Coach." Josie also started a card campaign with people from all over the United States, and our mailman started to look a bit haggard. Neighbor Jackie took over the role of "Support Coordinator." She organized the "meals on wheels" effort, a pre- and postchemo party at the gym, and numerous other events. She and two other friends, Sandi and Diane, also served as "Fitness Coaches," making sure Ann stuck to her gym routine. Ann never had time to feel sorry for herself, as friends always dragged her off to

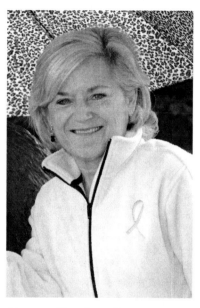

exercise or called if she wasn't at one of her regular classes. I can't say enough good things about being physically sound as you go through this. The operation and the chemo really knock you down, and you will need good physical resilience to carry through. Patty in Boulder became Ann's "Holistic Healing Coach." On a regular basis, she remotely provided Reiki, a form of energy healing, to Ann. She also sent special music for her to play and unique handmade gifts, such as a medicine bag, healing bracelet, and affirmation cards.

Cancer Coach —Jo.

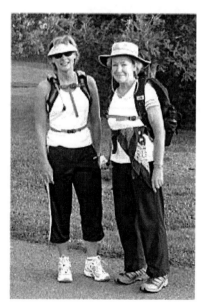

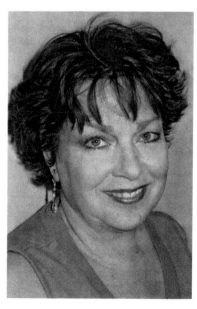

Walking strong with Coach Jackie.

Holistic Healing Coach—Patty.

Ann had joined a local gym called Cross Court, and, as we went through this process, the members there entered our lives. What was it with those people anyway? They all started wearing pink and decided that Ann needed food. I viewed this effort with a large dose of skepticism until "meals on wheels" got into production. Unbelievable! It was all edible, go figure! When you added the neighbor's contributions, it's a wonder we didn't blimp-up big-time. I guess what saved us was that everyone's mind runs to form, given our backgrounds. If someone's sick, give em' soup! Damn, I like soup, but if I don't see any for awhile it'll be just fine.

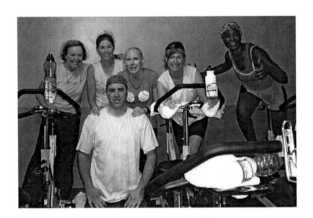

Cross Court gym friends sporting pink. (left to right) Jackie, Betsy, Fire Chief Drew, Annie, Sandi, and Diane.

Perhaps one of the funniest Cross Court stories involved Drew, the gym manager, who was also the local town fire chief. At 6 feet 7 inches, Drew is a manly man. In support of Ann, he wore a pink T-shirt and bandana when teaching Ann's Tuesday morning Spin Class. One of his firemen caught him in the act and reported the so-called feminine wear to the other firefighters. They commenced teasing, like a bunch of rabid dogs, until Drew explained why he was wearing pink. The crew quickly turned on the tattletale, and Drew became a firehouse hero.

Over ten women from the gym and neighborhood formed what they called "Annie's Team." In addition to exercise, they got involved in other activities. One was coordinating a 5K walk in the local "Oxford Day" celebration. The event was sponsored by an organization called Women Supporting Women that provides help to those with breast cancer. It was a way for Ann and the group to reach out in support of other women with breast cancer. And, before I knew it, they roped me into soliciting businesses to sponsor the event. Figure that! I was the very one that initially had wondered why women needed such support groups.

Amidst all this wonderful support, I received the crowning blow. When Ann embarked on the chemo trail, I was informed after the first treatment that subsequent visits would be handled by Jackie and Sandi. I was not needed …thank you very much! All I will say about this is that each session required several hours. Ann took a book each time, which never got cracked. What in the world did these women talk about? Even given my limited exposure (I insisted on going to more than one session anyway), it was sad to see those who came for treatment by themselves. You need a hand to hold or a shoulder to lean on while going through this. Do not let fair maiden do this on her own!

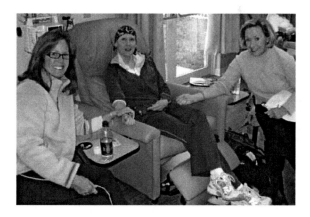

Sandi and Jackie glad they aren't getting the magic juice.

39

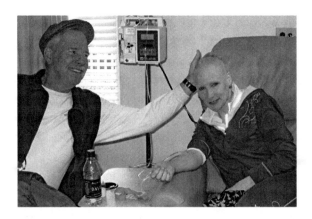

Bald is beautiful.

Lastly, whoever provides your support, tell them thank you. Say it loud and often! People just want to know that their efforts are meaningful. They certainly were for us. **A very special "thank you" to our entire support team! You were kick ass!**

CHAPTER 10

General Tips for Partners

Okay, what follows are a few partner tips to help you both through the daily process. These worked for us, so hopefully you will also find value in them. Some may come naturally, while others will be a struggle and require extra effort.

Laughter—I contend that there needs to be as much of this as you can muster. Personally, I've found humor in almost everything in life. More often than not, in my own absurd or predictable reactions to things. Being a basic dumb-ass does provide comic relief to others, and in the case of cancer, can relieve tension immediately. If you have the cojones to share all the stupid things you are going to do during this time, my bet is you'll get more than a chuckle or two. I'm not big on cancer humor per se, although it may have its place. However, I'd be careful, as some people, including others with cancer, may find it inappropriate. My advice is to make sure you know your audience when joking. Having some levity in conversations is great and can help people become more comfortable talking about the situation. But too much humor, or wrongly timed, can have the opposite effect.

Exercise—Your partner's body is going through a lot, and she will likely be pooped. Moderate exercise can help her recover from the effects of treatment. It can help her restore strength, maintain bone density, reduce fatigue, control weight, and boost her mood. So encourage your partner to exercise. Even if we are talking casual walks, do something to get the blood moving and the body out of the wait-and-see mode. There are so many important things to think about, but this one will help her tackle the mental and physical challenges in ways I can't describe. Be her coach—don't take "no" for an answer.

Hydrate, Hydrate, Hydrate—You've got to be a force in this activity. This is especially true shortly after chemo treatments when nausea is likely to be present. Think about it. When you're nauseous, you don't want anything upsetting the proverbial apple cart, so drinking water or apple juice would be like calling the IRS and asking for an audit. I have to believe that self-inflicted pain is only appealing to a small segment of our society, so drinking fluids will not be high on your partner's to-do list right after chemo treatments. Enter water boy. You have to encourage, plead, and do whatever (short of medieval torture techniques) to get water and fluids into your partner's system. The practical implication here is that you want to flush the system of these chemicals as soon as possible. The quicker they are out, the sooner the patient returns to normal. And believe me, you both want this to happen quickly. Drinking at least six to eight glasses of water-based liquid the day before, day of, and day after chemo is recommended. Actually, drinking this much water every day is always prudent, even for healthy people.

Ambiance—Creating the right ambiance postsurgery and during chemo or radiation is very important. You need to be thoughtful in creating the right atmosphere. Try putting on some soft background music. Open the blinds and let the sun come in and cheer up a room. If it's chilly, start a fire and get a cozy blanket for her. Close the blinds or drapes in the evening and put on soft lighting. Try to create an environment that is conducive to healing and comfort.

Nests—Beware of the nests! Women are inherent nesters. It's in their DNA. Think of your home. It's likely her nest and put together to be comfortable, warm and friendly. When your partner goes through this cancer ordeal, the nesting urge really comes out. They try to create mini-nests where they feel comfortable and secure. It makes them feel good or, at least better. Your bedroom is a likely candidate for this, more so than normal. Best bet is to leave them alone. You can straighten up a bit but putting everything back to its normal spot will likely get you dirty looks, or worse.

Ann's major nest was in the bedroom. It was filled with cards, flowers, balloons, a pink feather boa and all manner of things meant to cheer her up. One day while in my helpful mode, I tried to do the right thing and approached the sagging balloons with the trash can in mind. Ann had a somewhat different opinion. "Touch those balloons and I'll break your arm!" This was clearly an exit-stage-right opportunity, so I beat a hasty retreat. The nests will take care of themselves over time, so just let them be.

Entertainment—Unless you are a stand-up comic with unlimited material, you are going to need some assistance in this area. The idea here is to let the patient go off into another world rather than be focused on how crappy she feels. Suggestion: buy a bunch of trashy magazines, then go to Blockbuster and get a stack of chick flicks. You'll know the former because the covers will have a bunch of Hollywood types or wannabes in varying states of undress, or declaring they've been wronged. The latter is obvious, as there is usually a man and a woman kissing on the cover or the title makes absolutely no sense.

Drugs Are Your Friend—This may offend some alternative medicine types, but if you are following normal protocols, it's true for the most part. Pain medicine is provided for a reason. If your partner has pain, then ask her to take it. If your partner has nausea, make sure she takes the anti-nausea stuff. Ann was suffering from nausea after her first chemo treatment, throwing up, and generally feeling rotten. I asked her about the anti-nausea meds and she said she had a few hours to go before she took the primary pill again. I asked about the additional anti-nausea meds we got and she said she had not yet tried them. I responded that she was the one going through this, so she could do as she saw fit, but if it were me, I'd be popping those babies like M&Ms. She took one pill and the world got better. "Don't be a hero" can be your only coaching around this. I mean, what's the point?

Having said this, drugs do have a downside. In particular, pain pills and chemo. They will clog you up worse than cat hair in a drain. The doctors say that if this happens, try a stool softener. The nurses will tell you it is going to happen. So, go get some Milk of Magnesia and just do it. Go with the nurses! And use it sooner versus later. Ann learned to take it about one day after chemo because she knew what was coming.

Chores—Every couple has chores divided up the way it seems to make sense to them. Well, that division will need some adjustment. Our experience went like this. At surgery and for a brief time thereafter, I did it all. Immediately after chemo and for a few days following, I did it all. As Ann started to feel better, she reasserted herself into the normal routine. I believe this is a natural, healthy response. The partner needs to take over at certain stages, then let the patient spread her wings under some supervision. Don't let them overdo it. Be ready to step in and assist on a moment's notice. For guys, this means you should do some, if not all the shopping. Do the laundry and ironing. Clean the kitchen, cook, run the vacuum cleaner, take out the trash, pay the bills, and so forth. I don't care how molly-coddled you've been up to this point, you have to step up and do what's right. When you are tired, sick, or not on your game, there is nothing more depressing than looking around and seeing a bunch of things that need to be done. Guys, get rid of those things, and let her concentrate on getting better, not taking care of you.

Nurses—I mentioned this before. Listen to them. They have practical knowledge about typical postsurgery, radiation, and chemo reactions. You get the real scoop in layman's terms, which, from a male perspective, means you actually understand.

Little Things Count—I've already talked about creating the right ambience. That is an example of little things counting. They make a difference and will be noticed. She'll know you are thinking of her and are giving it your best. So look around and see what you can do.

Here's one that really got it done. During chemo, Ann often suffered night sweats (chemo brought on menopause) and felt completely rung-out the next day. So, I'd draw her a bath or she'd do it herself. While she was engaged, I'd put fresh sheets on the bed and fluff her pillows. Often the bath would take all her energy, but when she crawled back in bed, she had fresh crispy linen. Man, when you are not feeling well, that's a very good feeling.

Caregiver Take Care— It's amazing how much this process takes out of the caregiver. Guys like to think they are tough and can handle anything, but frankly, we are not as good as women when it comes to flexibility and adapting. Guys, take care! You are going to need time off. Get it when you can and don't miss opportunities to relax. When she gets tired and takes a nap, take one, as well, if it's needed. If she's feeling good, then go play golf, go fishing or hunting, drink a beer with the boys, read a book, or whatever. Just do it! You are no good to your loved one if you get run-down or sick. Who the hell cares if you don't feel good? Well, you should, even if no one else does, because you're in this for the long run. You are of no value if you can't help your partner reach the finish line. So, do whatever is necessary to keep fresh and be the game breaker. Do you want to be the MVP or one of those who left the gate strong but faltered in the end?

However, I will say this. Do these things carefully. You may need to suspend some pre-planned activities such as out-of-town trips, etc. Take it on the fly when opportunity presents itself, but pre-planned events have a way of making uncomfortable choices. Avoid them!

Ask for Help—If you've got kids in the house or are still working, dealing with cancer will be harder yet! But, (Isn't there always a but?) ask for help. Get the kids involved and ask for their help. Think about when you were young. What did you want? To be treated as an adult? To have someone count on you? To be needed? To make a difference? I'd wager money!

As to working, I don't think one should use their job or breadwinner role as an excuse to avoid the burden of supporting your partner during this time. I was in corporate America over thirty years and all you have to do is ask for help. Men don't like to do this because it makes us vulnerable and something less than invincible (another one of those gender differences). But what's more important, your fragile ego or your partner's welfare? There can be lots of tension in this one. You can balance both but only with some honesty about yourself and what's going on.

The truth is…most meetings you just "can't" miss are crap. The status quo usually remains by dealing with a few action items. The truth is…we don't want anyone to think they can do without us. The truth is…there is always someone who wants our position/job. The truth is… 99.9 percent of the people you are working for will respect your attempts to balance family and business during something like cancer. The other 0.1 percent you shouldn't be working with anyway. That's the truth! The truth is…you are an adult and get to make a choice!

Are you still hanging in there? Good! I hate to get preachy on you, but balance is only difficult if you are out of touch with where the heavier weight lays. Too abstract? Okay—then let's try this…some things are more essential than others. What is most important to you?

CHAPTER 11

Hair – Going Au Naturel

HAIR. Hair, or rather the lack thereof, is a big problem. Your partner is likely going to lose her mane if she is doing chemo. If she's taking Adriamycin there may be a one-in-a-million chance that she won't lose her hair, but it's a rare result. As one oncologist told us (verified by one of the all-knowing nurses), get over it and get your head around it.

Hair loss occurs because chemotherapy targets all rapidly dividing cells—healthy cells, as well as cancer cells. Hair follicles are structures in the skin filled with tiny blood vessels. Hair is formed by some of the fastest growing cells in the body, but as the chemo does its work against cancer cells, it also destroys the healthy hair cells. That's just the way it is—you get the good with the bad. Some chemotherapy drugs affect only the hair on your head. Others cause the loss of eyebrows, eyelashes, pubic hair, and hair on your legs, arms, or underarms.

Most guys lose some of, if not all, their hair as they get older. So to us it's just the natural order of things. Well, there are those with the flop-over dos to contend with, but they seem to be in the minority. Women losing hair though, this is a big deal. Just think of all the time they spend messing with it. They arguably spend this time so they can look nice for us, and we thank them for it. But the truth is, it's more than that. Hair for a woman sort of defines her. She is hardwired to care for it to the extreme. In a nutshell, she is ONE with her hair. So losing this extension of herself is extremely emotional. It's like having your ego smashed big-time.

So how can the ever-sensitive male deal with this event while his partner suffers the pangs of going bald? I have not a clue! I only know what I did, and I'm not sure it was right or would be appropriate for everyone. I only knew that I had to do something. I'm convinced that the worst thing you can do is ignore what's going on or try to blow it off as no big deal. So, if I wasn't going to ignore it, I decided to make an event out of it.

Ann's hair started coming out after the second chemo treatment (the timing was pretty typical, according to the oncologist). As luck would have it, two of her sisters, Janis and Amy, had come out to be with her. So, we had a built-in audience for the shearing. We got the camera out and broke open a bottle of wine. Using the hair trimmers from my electric razor, I went to work. We saw a Mohawk, punk, and other styles as we proceeded. We tried to put as much humor and levity into the situation as we could. Her sisters were magnificent! I'm not sure how it would have gone without them. As it was, we still had plenty of sad looks but Ann was never allowed to go into a shell and feel alone. We were there for her.

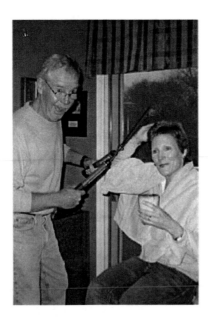

Looks easier in the barber shop!

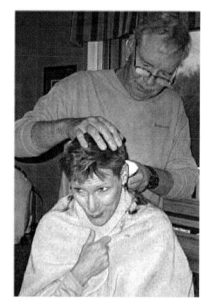
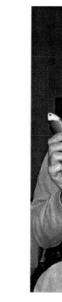

Need a clip?   **Did I take too much?**

At this point, your options are a bit limited if you are going to cover up old baldy. Some women probably don't bother, but I think you'd freeze to death with that choice. Bear in mind this insight is from a man whose hair is thinning and wears hats all the time.

Wigs— Wigs are a popular option. Heck, our medical provider even covered most of the cost. Ann got a couple of synthetic wigs, but there are also those made from real hair if your checkbook can afford it. My suggestion is that if you have one nearby, go to a wig shop that regularly deals with cancer patients, as they create a more supportive experience.

The wig process surprised me. When we entered a wig shop for cancer patients, there were no guys around. Now what's that all about? Why weren't partners there to be supportive? My advice is to be there, if at all possible. You need to be engaged in every aspect of this.

In our case, the women in the shop were very hushed, as they silently moved in and out of private sitting areas. The manager was by herself and said all the fitting rooms were occupied. We said this wasn't a problem—we'd just nose around and try on the wares at the nearest mirror. I started yanking wigs down and Ann put them on. Some of them were so absurd that we started laughing and carrying on. Women suddenly appeared from the sitting rooms. One lady, in particular, kept coming back with the same wig on after trying something different. Ann glanced over at her and told her it really looked nice. She glanced at me, and I said it looked nice, as well. She responded that everyone liked it except her mother. I laughed and said, "Hell, when's the last time you ever listened to her?" She said, "You're right! And she's sitting right over there." The room erupted in laughter as old stone face gave me the evil eye! There was a lot of chatter and sharing by the women after that. You really need to take this task on boldly and not be embarrassed.

However, there can be a few set-backs in this process. For example, Ann was wearing a wig, when our granddaughters asked to see under it. Ann had tried to prepare the girls for this moment. So, Ann ripped off the wig and Kylie, the younger one, immediately said "Annie put your hair back on. Please!" We absolutely laughed ourselves silly. Pure minds are a delight to see. There are so few!

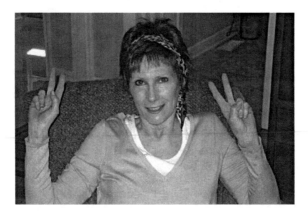

Wigs work!

Hats/Scarves/ Do-rags— All sorts of soft hats are out there for use. Ann got a bunch and they looked great! Scarves are also pretty effective and a lot more comfortable than a wig, according to Ann. However, do-rags were the real McCoy. Ann found an old Harley

Davidson do-rag out in the yard that the dogs had liberated from a garage basket filled with hats, etc. She washed it and one morning I heard her giggling in the bathroom. Sure enough, she had it on and WOW! All she needed were some leather pants and black boots. She tried it out at the gym and loved it. Having the Internet at her disposal, she ordered every color under the sun and then some. She discovered that they were comfortable at night, kept her head warm, and didn't slip off. They were great, and she was constantly getting unsolicited compliments from both men and women about her head gear (including people who didn't know she had cancer).

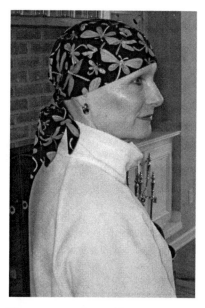

Do-rags preferred!

In summary, BALD is BEAUTIFUL. Guys need to be supportive and complimentary as their loved one keeps trying to look good for them...even without hair. You might also see the "no-eyebrows-or-eyelashes" look as you go down the chemo path. This one is a bit more problematic if your mate wears glasses and struggles to draw them on. But, what's a wavy line or two between friends? Count your blessings that she's still with you.

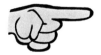

PARTNER TIPS

Know What to Expect—The degree of hair loss depends on the particular chemo drugs used. For example, Adriamycin causes complete hair loss on the head, usually during the first few weeks of treatment. Some women also lose eyelashes and eyebrows. Cytoxan causes minimal hair loss in most women, but some may lose a great deal. Taxol often results in significant hair loss from the head, brows, lashes, pubic area, legs, and arms.

Hair Growth—Her second biggest question after, "Will my hair fall out?" is "When will my hair grow back?" The answer depends on the treatment. If your partner has chemotherapy, here's a typical timetable for hair growth:

> Two to three weeks after chemotherapy ends—a baby soft fuzz emerges (Ann's started growing during chemo with Taxotere)
>
> One month after—real hair starts to grow at its normal rate
>
> Two months after—an inch of hair

How long it takes to grow back a full head of hair (and pubic hair, lashes, and brows, if she lost them too) varies from person to person. Generally, the hair most likely to fall out is the hair that tends to grow back the fastest. That means hair on the top of the head grows faster than eyebrows or eyelashes.

Like A Baby—The nurses described the hair growth process to be "like a baby's." Many women get curls, just like new babies. Over time, with hair cuts and growth, the curls settle down or disappear altogether. In general, the message is that hair may come in different than it went out.

Go With the Flow—Be prepared for lots of new looks and surprises as the hair transition takes place. In addition to the curls and general texture change, the color can change. Ann had colored her hair for years and didn't know what to expect. It came in silver-gray with some pepper. So, off she went to have it colored. She discovered that the color didn't take as well as before chemo. She ended up with what she termed "poop brown" hair, which she immediately changed again within a week. At this point I started to lose it. For crying out loud, she had hair. Who the hell cared what color it was or how many curls there were? Well, stop the presses. Guess who this was about? Once again, I had to hit the pause button. I wondered how many times I'd need to learn the same thing over again. Damn, there was a similarity to golf in this somewhere.

Loaner Wigs—If you can't or don't want to spend the money for a wig, check out the local American Cancer Society. They often have what is referred to as a wig salon, where you can borrow wigs. To find your closest ACS location, go to www.cancer.org.

Look Good, Feel Better Program—This is a free non-medical, brand-neutral national public service to help women offset appearance-related changes from cancer treatment. The session provides a hands-on workshop including a skin care/make-up application lesson, demonstration of options for dealing with hair loss, and nail care techniques. The programs are organized by the American Cancer Society. More information can be found at www.lookgoodfeelbetter.org.

CHAPTER 12

Sous Chef Partners

Let's start with a basic premise: If you don't feel like eating, then you sure as hell don't feel like cooking. The translation for this is that the guy needs to step up and takeover. When Ann was on chemo every two weeks, I found that her appetite and desire to prepare meals were much improved in week two over week one. So, I tended to takeover week one and assist in week two.

Cooking has never bothered me. I always figured if you blew it bad there was takeout somewhere. Plus, when I retired and Ann kept working, 75 percent of the cooking duties shifted to me. For others, this shifting of cooking duties may seem a daunting task. Some old-school guys have never cooked a day in their lives. Well, it's time to break that barrier, and it's significantly easier than you think.

First of all, I'm not a nutritionist. If you want really good advice, ask your doctor or see a specialist. We did find some useful information on how to get nutrition during cancer treatment on a Mayo Clinic Web site. Some of their ideas are included below in Partner Tips, but it's worth looking at the full list. Go to: www.mayoclinic.com/ health/cancer/HQ01134 .

I only know what worked for us, but what may work for you is likely different to some extent. Don't be afraid to experiment a bit. Besides, your pathetic attempts to cook will probably create a lot of humor for someone who needs it. Look at this as a two-for-one opportunity.

PARTNER TIPS

The Microwave Is Your Friend—Cardinal rule number one (and maybe the most important) is that the MICROWAVE IS YOUR FRIEND! I suggest you get up immediately and go kiss this appliance. It's going to save your butt during this adventure into meal preparation. Let's assume that friends, neighbors and relatives are going to take pity on you and prepare some meals for your eating pleasure. Now, this will be more about them wanting to ensure that your spouse gets proper nourishment than trying to help you, but you do get the side benefits, in any event.

While some of these meals are served cold, I'll bet the majority will need to be heated, particularly since you are likely to get soup, the standard 'get better' food. You always have the stove top and oven as alternatives, but when you can heat something up in the serving dish, it seems to me that you've just saved washing pots and pans (and they say guys aren't clever).

Now to the microwave. Guess what? All those numbers are on there for a reason. It gives you the chance to get something hot without overcooking it. So here's what I usually do. Let's use soup as an example, but it works with most everything. Put a bowl of soup in and put the timer on three minutes and the power on Level 3. This gets you going in the right direction and is helpful to bring refrigerated items to room temperature. Then zap it again for one to one-and-a-half minutes on Level 4 then give it a taste. Serve or zap it for another minute on Level 5. The key here is to bring the temperature up gradually so you maintain taste and don't overcook the meal. I've used this technique for everything imaginable, and it's easy as pie. I suppose you could always go to the microwave cookbook if you were industrious, but I've never read it and I probably won't.

Leftovers Are Your Friend—Cardinal rule number two has to be that LEFTOVERS ARE YOUR FRIEND. Anytime you actually cook, you need to think about two meals. What can I initially cook that will provide another meal in a couple of days? That is the question to be answered. With your new-found reheating skills you kill two birds with one stone. Besides, it makes meal planning twice as easy. If you're still working or have kids to feed in addition to your partner, this is the only sane mindset to have.

Be Flexible—Cardinal rule number three is to BE FLEXIBLE AND CREATIVE. Your spouse/partner's tastes are going to be out-of-whack, so go with whatever sounds good to her. And believe me, her tastes will be all over the place and change frequently. Think about adding more flavor than you might normally use to perk the food up. Chemo impacts taste buds and leaves a funny taste in the mouth, so you want to overcome that as much as you can. Your new friends are Tabasco, Lea & Perrin, BBQ sauce, and teriyaki. Use the dickens out of spices, as well. My favorites are garlic powder, onion salt, pepper, and any of the Paul Prudhomme spices. Flavor it up. You'd better taste the dishes donated by friends, as well. Most need spicing up because the cooks naturally assume that sick people require bland foods. They just don't realize that chemo messes with taste buds.

Other Tips
— If your partner doesn't feel like eating much, try giving her small amounts more frequently.
— Limit fluids during meals, as they can fill your partner up to the point she doesn't eat the more nourishing food.
— Limited consumption of alcohol is recommended, but a small amount of wine or beer before meals may stimulate her appetite. (Yes, this came from Mayo Clinic!)
— Keep snacks readily available—cheese, nuts, peanut butter, crackers, etc.
— Cold or room temperature foods may be more appealing, particularly if strong smells are bothersome.
— Be careful with uncooked fruits and vegetables. They can harbor harmful bacteria and should   be washed for thirty to sixty seconds before ingesting. Try to avoid these foods when dining out to minimize the risk of infection.
— Limit refined sugar, as some studies have found a connection between sugar and cancer.
— Keep some hard candies around to help your partner with the bad taste in her mouth. Ann likes Baskin-Robbins Hard Candy— only ten calories each and better for teeth.

In the next chapter, I have included a few fail-safe recipes that I like and Ann tolerates. Hope they help!

CHAPTER 13

Recipes for the Inexperienced

Before we get started, let's get real. You don't have to cook all that much if you are of a mind not to. You likely have access to every fast food joint known to man. Then there is the deli section at the grocery that usually does some kind of prepared meal, and you have the frozen food section to choose from, as well. Frankly, not wanting to pork-up, we have limited our access to fast food, but I've always liked our cooking over the other options. For example, the smell of chicken roasting at the grocery is typically better than the taste. However, that's us, and maybe it's not you. For that matter, your choices may be limited due to kids or job responsibilities. Do the best you can, but you need to take on this responsibility.

Dining Postsurgery—If surgery is involved, like a mastectomy, this is pretty simple from a food standpoint. Lots of fluids, start slow, and build up. This is about serving somewhat bland foods early on that are easy to consume. Then you build to more substantive fare. You should have been there and done that in some form or fashion with other illnesses.

Dining Postchemotherapy—This is a different animal altogether. For us, the chemo every two weeks took on a pattern. It was start slow and build over the next two weeks, then redo the process. So, if we are in day one, two, or three after chemo, what worked were saltine crackers, cottage cheese, and apple sauce. Ice cream was appealing, but with the cautions around refined sugar. Ann did the sugar free ice cream bars. Of course, drink lots of water or other fluids like apple juice. This is a very difficult time, as nausea is at its height and the smell of pizza throughout the house is likely to upset the apple cart. So, you have to be somewhat sensitive to odors early in the cycle. The other realization we had was that we started out bland and then spiced things up during the cycle. You want to be a bit of an irritant during all this. No matter how much food or fluid intake she has, it's never quite enough. Always encourage one more bite or drink…it will pay dividends.

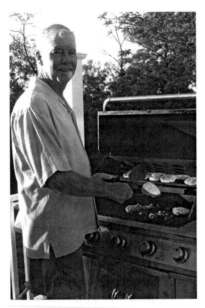

Chef Bob works his magic!

Following are recipes we like that I can handle. Nothing very fancy! They require a moderate effort and usually have a bias toward leftovers:

SALMON STEAKS/FILETS

This works with almost any fish, we just happen to like salmon. Get a glass or ceramic dish, spray with Pam and put the filets in it. Put some Chef Paul Prudhomme's Magic Seasoning Blends—Seafood Magic on the fish or use Tony Chachere's Original Creole Seasoning. Also sprinkle some garlic powder/salt and onion powder/salt. Cut up a lemon and squeeze the juice on the fish. Then put butter or margarine slices on top of the salmon. You're ready to rock! Put the oven on about 300 degrees and cook for about twenty to thirty minutes. The real key here is that most people cook fish like their mother cooked a roast. This is wrong. You want it cooked but tasty and moist. Feel free to check the fish as often as necessary. When it looks done, it usually is.

SURPRISE CASSEROLE

Now, everybody has one of these floating around. I like mine because I like noodles and mushroom soup and flexibility. My mother made this, but she always threw in a can of tuna. I find canned tuna very acceptable for cats and marginally so for humans, but that's a personal bias. I'm sure you have your own.

Okay, locate a casserole dish. This dish will give itself up because it is usually round and three to four inches deep. Pam that baby up! Here's the hard part…find some egg noodles. If they are dry, then boil them in water until they start to soften. If you are really clever and found the ones in the store that are soft and don't need boiling, then just throw the noodles in the casserole dish—that's the round thing you found earlier. Open a can of mushroom soup and dump most, if not all, of it in the dish with the noodles. Do the water or milk thing that is suggested on the can.

Now you can get clever. I don't think Mom ever tumbled to this concept. You can put just about anything you want into this goop. Tuna, any fish, sausage (pre-cooked), ham, chicken, etc…just go crazy, it all works. The meat, if any, needs to be pre-cooked or from some of your leftover stash in the frig.

Add spices if you are feeling frisky, then stir it all up. Most people would use a spoon here, but whatever works for you is fine. Now put cheese on top. Personally, I prefer Velveeta! Probably the worse stuff in the world, but I love it because it tastes so good. Layer slices of this, or whatever, on top of the goop. Set oven to 350 degrees. Give it forty-five to fifty minutes of cooking and you are in business. The key here is when the cheese starts to darken up, you are pretty much ready to go. Take it out and let it set for five minutes.

PORK CHOPS

This is the other white meat, if you have not heard. Filets or chops, the recipe is the same.

Get the meat to room temp. Then stab it with a fork or knife. Season up with Chef Paul Prudhomme's Magic Seasoning Blends-Meat Magic or Tony's Chachere's Original Creole Seasoning and add garlic and onion seasonings. Here comes the hard part; lather both sides with Italian salad dressing. Pick what you like, but the brand by Paul Newman worked for us. You need to let this marinate for an hour or two (in the frig or out, take your pick).

Throw these puppies into a glass or ceramic dish that you have Pammed-up previously, and put them into the oven that you have preheated to 375 degrees. The key to this meat is a lot like chicken. You want it cooked but not dried out.

Give it about forty minutes or so and check on the progress. When you see just a little pink, turn off the oven and serve everything together. A little pink is okay, because the meat will continue to cook in the turned-off oven or on a plate as you gather up other items for dinner. This meal goes well with rice. Somebody is going to love you!

SPLIT PEA SOUP

This is easy but a bit time-consuming. Get a 16 oz. package of split peas and wash/drain them. Put peas in a large pan with 6 or so cups of water. Add about 2-3 cups of canned chicken broth. Throw in a couple of ham hocks, which will add taste to the broth as it cooks. Add carrots (you can buy a bag of the baby sized ones and avoid having to peel and cut them up). Dice one to two onions and put them in the pot. Bring everything to a boil and then simmer. During the simmer time, generously add spices to taste, including salt, pepper, garlic and onion powder. Dice up some pre-cooked ham (buy a big chunk, not slices) and throw it in the mix. I often add half a bag of lentils if I determine the soup needs more thickening. How long the soup simmers just depends on how thick you like your soup, but it will take at least an hour. Remove the meat from the ham hock bones and return it to the soup before serving. If you're really industrious, buy a box of "JIFFY" Corn Muffin Mix and make muffins to go with the soup. Delicious!

STEAK

We don't eat it all that often, so we go with either filets or rib-eyes. Bring the meat to room temp and put your favorite seasonings on both sides. Or use my personal favorite, mesquite. Now the key to this one is how thick the meat is. Ann likes her meat medium, and I like mine rare. So I cook hers a minute on each side, searing, then throw mine on for two minutes a side while continuing to cook hers. The whole thing takes about six minutes, and we're both happy. The seasonings? For the most part they've cooked off but leave a great flavor. This meal usually worked in week two, just before the new chemo was due. It's good for the red blood cell count too.

CHEESEBURGERS/HAMBURGERS

For whatever reason, on day two or three after the initial chemo, the first real food that appealed to Ann was a cheeseburger. This worked for me, so I got into it. The key here is to be a bit creative. Let's assume you have ground beef or ground round that measures a pound to two pounds. Throw it in a bowl and crack an egg (raw) into the mess. Add spices like, garlic, onion and whatever. Now come the choices that the partner prefers. For us, it goes like this...

Put cubed cheese, onion and mushrooms into the mix. Put your hands in, squeeze it all together and make it into patties. I love grilling them because it is so easy. Here's a surefire way to grill and always have meat come out the way you want. If it's a gas grill, heat it up as hot as it will go. If using charcoal, you want to see a lot of white coals. The key here is to sear the meat on both sides, and it does not make a hoot what kind of meat it is. Do not listen to your wife or mother-in-law about all the bad stuff in meat. Personally, I'm not sure it's there, but if it is, you will cook it all away while actually retaining the original flavor, and it will be moist, unless over-cooked, of course. So, back to this searing thing. With hamburgers, it's about two minutes per side, then turn down the heat to halfway or, in the case of charcoal, close the vent. Another two minutes per side and you should be good to go, depending upon how thick you made those bad boys. The burgers should come out about medium. Kill the heat, slap a slice of cheese on top, close the lid and take out in about thirty seconds.

When dealing with beef, if you are stupid enough to ask how people want their meat, you will get responses of rare, medium rare, medium but with pink, medium with no pink, well, really well and a few I've forgotten. This is like people going to Starbucks and ordering coffee. Diet this and low-fat that and organic whatever. Forget all that crap. There are only three grades if YOU are cooking: done, pink and red. This is not hard and only requires that you wear a watch. Time what you are doing, and all is well. Key point is if the meat looks done on the grill, you have just likely over-cooked it. Why, you say? Because meat keeps cooking until it starts to cool down, ergo, when you think it needs another minute, take it off and take it in. By the time it hits the table you are good to go. If you blow it? Not to worry. Nuke it for thirty seconds on high in your old friend the microwave.

BBQ RIBS/CHICKEN

You may cringe at this, but the best way to cook these is just like steak and hamburgers. Initially sear the meat on each side for about two minutes. Then turn the heat down and lather with sauce, turning the meat every few minutes until done. Ribs can be pork or beef. If grilling chicken, it should be skinned. Only eat chicken with its skin once a year when you indulge and go to KFC or Popeyes. That's a health tip, but from a practical standpoint, when on a hot grill the fat in chicken skin flames and burns...a barbecuer's greatest fear.

SAUCE FOR BBQ

Use whatever you want, just keep in mind that immediately following chemo, less is best. Later, more is better (two-week cycle).

I can't believe I'm going to share with the world my particular BBQ concoction. I do this to let the male chefs know that you need not be held hostage to the supermarket choices, which are extensive and varied. If you find one you like, then go for it. My dad used to make his from scratch, and it would bring tears to your eyes if you got any whiff of what was going on in the kitchen. It was, however, the best I've ever had, bar none. The old dog did not share it with me, in part because it was different every time he made it. Oh well, us wannabes just keep trying. Here's what works for me...

Start with a bottle of Kraft Original Barbecue Sauce. Mix with the following ingredients: Tabasco sauce, Lea & Perrins, Soy or teriyaki sauce, fresh horseradish (it's usually where you find fresh fish in the grocery), and minced garlic. Then put a spoonful of French's Classic Yellow Mustard and the same amount of Colman's Mustard. Mix it all up and taste away. You get a real nice tangy sauce. For the two of us, we usually use half a bottle of Kraft's, several shakes of the liquids, and teaspoonfuls of the rest. The easy thing about doing this is you can add anything you want and leave out whatever doesn't appeal.

RED BEANS and RICE

We probably like this due to our stay in New Orleans, but it's a poor substitute for the real stuff. Anyway, get a box of Zatarain's Red Beans and Rice Mix and follow the instructions. When it's close to done, slice up some pre-cooked turkey sausage and mix it in. When everything is warm, throw on some Tabasco and go for it.

SIDES

Do whatever is appealing, but Ann likes Tater Tots or fries with her hamburgers. All you need is a flat cookie sheet and an oven. Baked potatoes are easiest if you nuke them (six to eight minutes) on high. Then there is Mac and Cheese, Rice-A-Roni, or white rice as substitutes. Veggies are good, and one of our favorites is steamed broccoli. Steam it until you can just get a fork through it, splash on some Italian salad dressing, and you'll be loved.

SALADS

We both love salads, but early in the two-week chemo cycle it was more apple sauce and cottage cheese with sliced apples/fruit added. We then moved on to green salads.

Start with the basics of lettuce. We like romaine and sometimes use the prepackaged mixed greens as well. Add tomatoes, sliced mushrooms, peppers, green onions, etc., in any combination. Remember the importance of really cleaning any raw vegetable to avoid the risk of bacteria.

Then, go for the spices—we really like McCormick Bon Appetit Seasoning Salt

Now for the fun! Here is a list of added ingredients we use. Rarely would they be used all together, but you can mix and match and get creative. Try these: hearts of palm, artichoke hearts, raisins, cranberries, almond slices, walnut pieces, cheese, tortilla strips, and croutons. Basically anything you find in the pantry that appeals to you will work. Have fun and experiment!

One other salad idea is to slice a head of iceberg lettuce into quarters, crumble some blue cheese over it, and add blue cheese dressing. Yummy! This salad is often served in fancy steakhouses so you'll feel like a real gourmet chef if you serve it.

═══

These are some of the basic meals that can get you through. They are nothing fancy but pretty easy to prepare. You may even start to like cooking, if you don't already. Find a good cookbook or two and go for it. Tip: your wife/partner has many stashed in the kitchen somewhere.

Remember, just trying to cook will do a lot for the spirits of the one you love. Besides, there's always takeout.

CHAPTER 14

Distractions

Distractions…let's talk about the concept briefly. Distractions are anything that takes the cancer patient's mind off the "Woe is Me" syndrome and feeling victimized. In part, I believe this gets the mental juices flowing, allowing the body to deal more freely with what's happening. Ergo, you can heal faster! This observation is without a medical degree or even consultation on my part. It's just anecdotal data.

What does a distraction look like? Let's start with visitors such as our daughters, Rhory and Rhiain, and our two granddaughters, Kari and Kylie. When they visit, there is a lot of noise, confusion and laughter. Sounds like a major distraction to me. They came as often as they could, as long as none were sick, and it was great. So, don't try to protect your loved one from others—they are better than medicine. The only caution here is to allow no "sickies" in. You are probably okay after a surgery like a lumpectomy or mastectomy, but chemo wipes out your white blood count and makes you susceptible to illness. Don't take the risk, even if it provides a needed distraction!

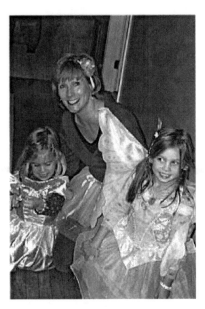

**Diversions abound with Kylie
and Kari.**

Relatives, in general, are a great source of distraction. In our case, all four of Ann's sisters came out to assist and be supportive. Your only responsibility in this is to be a scheduler. You need to monitor what your partner is going through and only schedule visitors when she is on the upswing. However, even this is only valid if you are always available to assist and care for someone when they are feeling like crap and need a little TLC. If your availability has limits, get as much help as you can. A good caregiver postsurgery and early in the chemo or radiation rounds is critical. The distractions are part of the healing process.

Additionally we had friends visit from Texas, Louisiana, The Netherlands and London, not to mention locals who just stopped by. The phone was forever ringing with people checking in and looking for updates. And, you know what? It was all magnificent! I love them all for their support and the distractions they created.

Perhaps the best part of all this is that nobody came or called without a story or a current problem. It was great! Ann grabbed onto these like Scotch Tape on paper. She went into a confidant, commiserate problem-solving mode. It was wonderful because while she did this, she was back to normal and the cancer was a forgotten thing. She worried over these things like a dog over a big bone. I couldn't have been happier! When these events happen for you, welcome them with open arms.

Don't assume that distractions are only of the two-legged variety. Animals can do wonders for the spirit. Case in point is the story of our dogs Maggy and Midnight.

We had decided to get a couple of dogs when we moved to Maryland, but we got busy and it didn't happen right away. Around July 2007, we were ready to start the pet search, but then Ann was diagnosed with cancer. I figured we'd put this off for a year, as we had other challenges to face. Apparently Annie had other thoughts. A week or two after her cancer diagnosis she asked, "What about the dogs?" I was thunderstruck by the question. After minimal discussion, it was apparent her mind was set. I was toast if this didn't come about. After twenty-five years of marriage you start to get a sense of the winds of inevitability blowing through and give it up sooner or later. I picked sooner!

Now this was a real experience. I thought you just went to the dog pound, found something, paid a couple of bucks, and brought it home. Well, pounds have become shelters, which include an adoption process. Has the world gone mad? Plus, these places are staffed by well-meaning, wannabe bureaucrats who only follow defined protocols and exercise no individual judgment. We found two dogs at the first place we went to, but Ann decided to check how child-friendly they were. So, she suggested I get in the kennel with them. I was damn near knocked down and pawed to death. On exiting, one dog escaped, so I went running after it. Ann thought this was fine sport. Ten minutes later and in a full-body sweat, I got the errant dog back in place and was filling out adoption papers. Upon submission and review, I was reminded that I checked the box that said these would be "outside dogs." The conversation then went like this:

"Yes, I did check that box."

"Well, we really like our adopted animals to be part of the family."

"Okay, I'm down with that."

"Yes, but you checked the 'outside' box. So, well we really …"
Then she repeats herself.

"I heard you the first time. What does that have to do with
whether they are part of the family?"

"We really…" She repeats herself yet again.

At this point I was starting to have an out-of-body experience.

She continues. "Well. I can't approve this. The director will have
to review it. She'll call you in a few days."

Great, obviously sanity will triumph and a more competent
bureaucrat will take charge. We waited by the phone with no call
back, so I assumed we were deemed unfit parents.

Determined that insanity should not prevail, we went to a shel-
ter in a neighboring county. As luck would have it, we found and res-
onated with two dogs (Lab mix—a brother and sister). All was cool.
We filled out the forms again and were told the director would call
back in a few days. Two days later, with no phone call, I went on the
offensive and called in. The director actually answered, and this is
what transpired:

"Yes, Mr. Musser, I was just looking over your application. I see
where you say these are going to be 'outside' dogs."

"That is correct."

"Well, we really like our adoptions to be part of the family."

Oh brother, this disease had permeated the whole of Maryland.
I started to wonder why they had the box to check if it is a given that
dogs can't be outside.

At that point, the conversation became a bit more spirited! In the
heat of battle, I explained that we had love in our hearts. We had an
invisible fence around the yard and had already bought several hundred dollars of supplies. I told her she seemed convinced that I was
going to chain the dogs to a tree and beat them once a day for good
measure.

She responded, "Well, we do like our adoptions…"

"Yeah, yeah, I got it the first time, and they will be, but just not
inside."

Her tone was now haughty. "Well, just how much of your yard
is actually fenced in?"

"How about eight acres!"

"Oh, well… where are they going to sleep?"

"In a garage."

She was persistent. "Does it have heat and A/C?"

This conversation was not going well, and I was losing it big-time. "These are bloody dogs, lady. They are not children. The garage has been insulated. It has a heater, and it has windows and fans."

"Well, we have this rule, but perhaps you are the exception."

I SHUT UP.

"When can you pick them up?"

It was the quickest flip-flop I ever saw. Ellen DeGeneres, where were you when I needed you?

This was a heck of a beginning, by all accounts, but the dogs were worth their weight in gold. This distraction brought much joy to our lives and theirs. Sixteen months old when we got them, Maggy weighed fifty pounds and Midnight tipped the scales at sixty. Eight months later (because the dogs were not part of the family) Maggy was a svelte seventy-five pounds and the bruiser was over ninety.

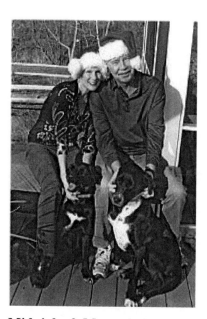

**Midnight & Maggy bring holi-
day cheer.**

There is no way to tell ahead of time what your distractions might be, but when they happen, go with the flow. This is, in large part, your partner's need to return to her normal mode of behavior. As protective as you might feel, you have to let it go but still monitor that it's under control. When she gets too tired or starts stressing, then you have to step in and make things go away. Jump too early and you're toast once again. There's a bit of a balancing act around this, but with a little sensitivity you can get it done correctly. Don't worry too much, as you are likely to blow it once or twice. When you do, fess up, laugh about it, and promise you'll do better in the future. This is unlikely, but who really cares? At least you're giving it your best!

CHAPTER 15

Bumps in the Road

Bumps in the road abound. It's amazing. You think you have the big issues covered and then a bump! Turns out, there are quite a few to deal with. But it's a lot like driving, grab the wheel and make an adjustment. You must remain fluid around these hurdles. You know your destination; you just have to make some small adjustments. In some respects, these changes are anticipated, but they are without conscious focus. When they show up, some can be big elephants in the room that nobody talks about. This is not a good idea. Keep the conversation going and be understanding. Laugh when you can. After all, it's just part of the process!

Below is a short explanation of some of the issues we faced and how we dealt with them.

Fatigue—If you're in the midst of breast cancer treatment, your body is in a war against cancer. It needs all its resources to fight the disease, so it shuts down your energy for other activities that would take away your strength from the battle. Fatigue is the result.

Ann found it a bit unpredictable, so it frustrated her not knowing when it would hit the hardest. In fact, fatigue lingered when treatment was over, as she was trying to catch up with everything she had put on the back burner. There's also no way to tell how long fatigue may last. The experts say that, as a rule of thumb, it takes at least as long as the amount of time from diagnosis through the end of treatment. So, for example, if diagnosis and surgery took two months, followed by six months of chemotherapy, the fatigue will likely take at least eight months to go away.

There are lots of ways to help address fatigue. Here are my tips: encourage catnaps, but beware of long naps or your partner may end up wide-awake in the middle of the night, wondering why she can't sleep. Explain the problem to others. Be up-front that fatigue is a significant side effect resulting from the treatment. Encourage your partner to ask for what is needed (e.g., flexibility or scheduling) to help her manage her low energy. Ask for help and accept the offers of goodwill from family and friends. Identify stressors such as job, family, or money. If you can, try to make it better. Support her in giving up unimportant, unfinished business and in setting priorities. Join her in some sort of physical activity to boost her energy. Extend your timeline. Due to the lingering effects of fatigue, be prepared to help out well after treatment ends.

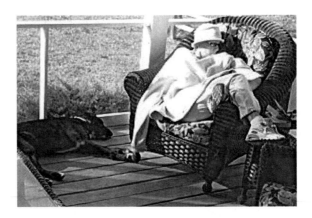

Even the dogs supported Annie's frequent naps.

Chemo Brain—The doctors and nurses mentioned this almost in passing. I guess they didn't want to scare us because it doesn't happen to everyone. But, if and when it happens, you and your partner will know it. For Ann, it started about at about the fourth chemo treatment.

Ann described this phenomenon as it was like her mind was in a fog—unable to concentrate, focus, and remember details. Research (yes, they have researched this) shows that what people are experiencing is called mild cognitive impairment, including the loss of the ability to remember certain things and complete tasks. The cause of the impairment during cancer treatment still isn't clear, nor is it understood how often it happens or what may trigger it. The doctors aren't sure what they can do about it, so you just have to deal with it! In fact, even though the term chemo brain implies a relation to chemotherapy, some say it isn't clear that chemotherapy is responsible. I assume they have not been through it because the connection was very clear to me.

Ann had a successful twenty-nine year career in the business world and was accustomed to being in charge. She had excellent planning, organization and delivery skills. She multitasked with the best of them by talking on the phone, cooking dinner, and working on a project all at the same time. So when chemo brain hit, it came as a bit of a shock and a major frustration. Some of the problems she noticed were as follows: struggling to find the right word, short-term memory lapses, inability to do her usual multi-tasking, and taking longer to finish tasks that were generally quick and easy. At points, she would elect not to drive any farther than the gym because of lack of focus. She's not the best driver anyway, so knowing she had chemo brain scared the crap out of me.

The subtleties of this are a killer! The truth is, witnessing chemo brain, you're going to think that you are the one losing it, like in the conversation below.

"Bob, we have to go see the doctor tomorrow."

"Okay, what time?

"12:40 PM."

"I thought we were going to the store tomorrow?"

"We are."

"I thought we normally saw the doctor on Tuesdays."

"Of course."

"Well, tomorrow is Monday."

"I know that! We're going to the store on Monday and the doctor on Tuesday!"

The moral to this story is that before you have a corrective conversation, consider that the moon and earth have both moved slightly out of orbit. Your mission is to be ready to go on Monday and Tuesday, whenever!

Some of your conversations will border on the absurd and some will leave you perplexed and wondering, "What did we just say?" The difficult part of this is just to understand what's going on. You can't make this better if you yell or become frustrated or even appeal to logic. It is what it is. It feels like your partner is having early dementia. You will find milk on the counter instead of in the refrigerator. You will find her car keys still in the ignition. She'll take twice as long as normal to do things. You have to remain patient and understanding. The craziness of it all may just lead you to drink early in the day.

Nausea and Vomiting—I have already touched upon this in other chapters, but it is such a big concern that it is worth saying a bit more. Most of us have grown up hearing stories of people who have had cancer and chemo made them very sick. This was one of Ann's biggest fears, to the extent that she felt sick even before the first couple of chemo sessions. However, what we experienced was that modern medicine has really progressed in addressing this problem. Vomiting can sometimes be prevented, and nausea can be reduced with medication. The key is to take the drugs prescribed by the doctor. Don't let your partner wait until she is experiencing problems. Stay ahead of the game!

Ann only vomited once, which was about thirty-six hours after her first chemo treatment. The oncologist had given her pills to take regularly and some "just in case" meds to take in between if she started to feel nauseous. She decided she would hold off for the regular pills. What a mistake, and one she only made once.

Nails—Just as hair is important to a woman's identity, so are her nails. That's why there is a nail salon on every other street corner in America. And, just as the chemotherapy affects hair because of its rapidly dividing hair follicle cells, so it affects nails. Nails may become pigmented or discolored. They may become more brittle and break more easily. Heck, the nail may actually lift off the nail bed. This can be a major disaster in some women's lives. Just don't let her panic. Remind her they will grow back.

As with the hair, let her know she is glamorous without those long sculptured nails, which can cause infection. She needs to clip those babies short and wear a nail strengthener. Hide her cuticle scissors or risk infection. And be a man; do the dishes. Excessive exposure to water can lead to fungal infection.

Menopause—At some point in every woman's life, her hormone production drops below the level required to continue her periods and menopause sets in. Ann was just moving into menopause and would normally have welcomed the end to monthly periods, bloating, and inconvenience. She could save money by not buying all the equipment that goes with the monthly cycle. However, her chemo brought on the sudden onset of full menopause at a time she was already dealing with a lot. So, the addition of hot flashes and mood swings wasn't all that welcome.

Actually, not all that welcome is an understatement! Thankfully, we have a king-sized bed but something more like a wrestling mat would have been more suitable. The covers were flying off and on more frequently than the Dow Jones' ups and downs and complicated by the fact that Ann is not known for subtle physical behaviors. I found myself waking up every couple of hours either freezing or roasting, as the covers came and went. Once I almost fussed at her, but common sense prevailed, and I grinned instead. The only question was—how long before I was let out of the clothes dryer that couldn't decide which cycle it was on? Sanity eventually prevailed, but it took a couple of months. If this happens to you, good luck! It will blow your socks off.

Mouth Sores—Just when you're not feeling great anyway, and your appetite is down, mouth sores (canker sores and ulcers) can raise their ugly heads. They are fairly common and can be a major irritant. Ann only had two small ones, which she attributed to closely following the nurse's prevention advice: 1) brush teeth two to three times daily with a soft toothbrush, 2) rinse regularly with a salt or baking soda concoction (six to eight times per day, especially after eating), and 3) avoid commercial mouthwashes. Ann kept a container with the magic juice right on her bathroom counter, as a constant reminder. The recipe is easy—mix one quart of water with three tablespoons of salt or baking soda.

Radiation Woes—Ann didn't have radiation, so this information is based on the experience of our friends who have gone through it. I'm adding this section because women who have had a lumpectomy generally follow with radiation, which significantly reduces the chance of reoccurrence.

Radiation does not hurt when it is administered. Nor does it cause nausea or hair loss. The side effects of radiation depend on the part of the body being treated. With breast cancer, most women experience a mild sunburn effect but severity can vary. Over-the-counter ointments and prescription creams are available to help with these problems and your doctor can advise what is best for your lady. Another major symptom is fatigue, which tends to worsen toward the end of the treatments.

CHAPTER 16

Intimacy

It's funny (or not) how such an important topic is rarely discussed by medical practitioners. About the only thing we were told was that we should avoid intercourse for forty-eight hours after chemotherapy. Yeah, like at ages sixty-four and fifty-three, the first thing we're going to do after chemo is jump in bed and go for it.

That said, many couples find that breast cancer diagnosis and treatment seriously disrupt their sexual lives. First, there are the most obvious issues for your partner—the physical changes, nausea, pain, empty energy reserves, emotional chaos, and that ever important self-image. Our society associates women's breasts with beauty, femininity, sexiness and motherhood. So, why wouldn't your partner feel threatened by breast cancer and its potential impact on intimacy? But, retaining intimacy in your relationship both during and after breast cancer is critical to overall recovery.

Like it or not, the cancer experience can strengthen or break a relationship. This is an opportunity, whether married or not, for you to show the depth of your love. It's like a test. When the going gets tough, will you really be there or will you bail? You need to remember that intimacy goes beyond sex. So, show lots of affection, as sex itself may not be on the table as often, at least initially.

Based on what we've read and our experience, communication is the key. After all, communication—talking and listening to each other—is important in any intimate relationship. This needs to start early on as you discuss treatment options—lumpectomy, mastectomy, reconstruction. And, it must continue during the entire healing process. This may not be an easy task for many men, but ask your partner about how she's feeling and concerns she has regarding being intimate. This is all a part of the think pink thing.

Once we talked, I was surprised to learn some of Ann's concerns, as they were big to her but not to me. For example: what should she wear, if anything, while being intimate? She was obviously somewhat self-conscious about the mastectomy. She hadn't been trying to hide her body from me, but intercourse would bring concerns up close and personal. She wondered if she should wear a wig or go *au naturel*. How would I react to no pubic hair? She set an Olympic record going through menopause and knew she'd have dryness not experienced previously, so we needed to deal with that. I had to laugh when she said she "felt like a virgin" in exploring each aspect of this new territory.

My advice? Talk, laugh, hold hands, experiment, take small steps as needed, and be patient. But most of all, show her you love every aspect of her—mind, spirit and body. Having her alive and well is what counts the most.

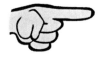 **PARTNER TIPS**

Give Up Mind Reading—It can only lead to problems. For example, you're thinking you are a sensitive, selfless guy willing to give up sex in support of your partner. So you quit talking about it, stop touching her, and, in general, discontinue making any flirtatious advances. She, on the other hand, interprets this as you don't find her sexy anymore. Big problem! Better to just talk about what is going on, and how the two of you want to address it.

Gifts—Give her things to feel feminine and sexy, like a new piece of lingerie. Or, if you are like me (not so comfortable buying such things), give her a gift certificate to her favorite store and encourage her to go shopping.

Body Changes—Surgery, chemo, and hormone therapy all take their toll on your partner's body. For example, women may experience a reduced sex drive, vaginal dryness, vaginal discharge, and/or pain at some point in the process. There are plenty of options for dealing with these—some prescription and some over the counter. Ask your doctor or the nurses for advice.

Timing Is Everything— We were told that if you stop being intimate altogether, it becomes more difficult to start up again. You may go through cycles where different forms of intimacy are more suitable (talking, touching, intercourse), but just don't go cold turkey. You'll only know what her needs are by keeping the line of communication open.

CHAPTER 17

Reconstruction

Finding out you have breast cancer is traumatic enough, but learning that you may lose one or both breasts is a double whammy. That's the way it happened with us on that memorable day, August 1, 2007. In the course of five minutes, the breast surgeon went from explaining Ann's breast cancer to recommending a mastectomy. She even suggested we consider a double mastectomy, although no cancer had been found in the right breast. Because lobular cancer has a slightly higher risk of spreading to the other breast, some women go ahead and have both removed. Talk about overload.

After getting a second opinion, we agreed a mastectomy of the left breast was the best course of action. Then we needed to make a series of decisions around reconstruction. How important was recreating the breast? Did she need surgical breast reconstruction to feel whole again? Some women elect not to reconstruct, but Ann wanted to do it. Next was which option to choose—implant or the use of one's own tissue? She chose an implant. Lastly, what about timing? The majority of women who are given the choice ask that the process for reconstruction be started immediately. For Ann, this meant putting in a temporary implant, called an expander, during the mastectomy.

About seventy-five percent of women who have mastectomies go on to have surgical reconstruction of one or both breasts. Roughly half of these women decide on artificial implants (saline or silicone). There has been a lot of controversy about the use of silicone-filled implants. They don't last forever, so be sure to ask about the lifespan of an implant. Silicone's advantage is that it is most like the normal breast in weight and consistency.

Artificial Implants—For most women, the skin that remains after mastectomy must be stretched or expanded to make room for the implant. To stretch the skin, the surgeon inserts a balloon-type device called a tissue expander under the chest muscle. The expander has a port (a metal or plastic plug or valve) that allows the surgeon to add increasing amounts of liquid over time (about six months) without extra surgery. Gradually, the skin and tissue are stretched to achieve the desired capacity. When stretching is achieved and the other treatments (e.g., chemotherapy) are completed, the expander is usually replaced with a permanent implant filled with either saline or silicone gel. Following this, the nipple reconstruction and areola tattooing can be done. Yes, you heard me right. They can make a nipple that looks pretty good.

Self-tissue Reconstruction—Another way to surgically reconstruct a breast is to take tissue from an area of your partner's body where she has extra to spare and move it to her chest. Skin, fat, and muscle is taken from the abdomen, back, or buttocks and used to make a new breast. One of these procedures is called the TRAM flap, meaning the flap comes from the transverse rectus abdominis muscle in the abdomen. It is an especially popular option for a woman with excess belly fat or an abdomen that has been stretched out by pregnancy, as a "tummy tuck" is essentially a fringe benefit of the surgery.

That gives you a general medical summary of options. Now, let me share how this went down with us in real life, as there were tears, laughter and near misses during this process.

The Tears—One of the few times that I saw Ann cry was about a week after she learned of her cancer. Her friend Jackie was returning from Africa, where she and daughter Wendy had climbed Mount Kilimanjaro. Ben, her husband, had invited us over for a welcome home drink. Ann decided to kill some time before we left and got on the Internet. She decided, without telling me, that it was time to check out pictures of women who had received reconstruction surgery. The next thing I knew, she came into the kitchen crying. In my ever-so-gentle way, I asked what was wrong, and she told me how awful the women looked after surgery. She was clearly horrified. I told her to get a hold of herself, as we needed to head to the Battaglinos. This was the second (and last) time I made the mistake of criticizing her tears. We took an extra ten minutes, talked a bit, agreed to ask the doctor for pictures, and then headed over to the affair.

As it turned out, when we went to Johns Hopkins Hospital, the nurse had a whole book full of pictures of women who had received reconstruction surgery—both implants and the flap procedures. We were amazed at how good they looked. Several were even more attractive postsurgery, largely due to the tummy tuck. My advice? Ask your doctor to see pictures. Don't jump on the Internet for this one.

The Laughter—Ann was very relieved when she awoke from surgery on September 20. She had a breast, or at least the start of one. When the drain came out a week later, she was able to pull on a top and go to a friend's birthday party looking fairly normal. A week after that, the expansions started and continued weekly until the chemo started October 23. On the days of expansion, we'd drive two hours to Johns Hopkins Hospital in Baltimore for a ten minute procedure that was relatively painless (until toward the end). But, what followed brought tears to our eyes—tears of laughter. That darn implant kept getting bigger, higher, and harder. Ann fondly named it Mount Kilimanjaro. She told me that if I heard her choking during the night, to roll over and check on her. She said she might be strangled by the expander! The other source of laughter was her trying to deal with the "lopsided look." I began to imitate her dilemma by putting my hands up under my shirt, with the left being much higher than the right. Anything for a laugh.

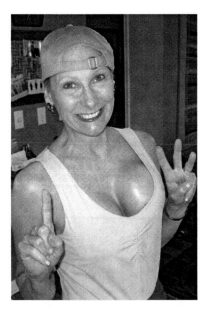

Mt. Kilimanjaro!

The Near Miss—So Ann has this metal plug under her skin, which was the port to the expander. They injected juice (saline) into it every week or two before chemo started. Somewhere in this process one of her doctors ordered an MRI. None of us connected the dots, so Ann went for the MRI at our local hospital and started talking to the technician about what was going on. The technician did one of those, "You got what, where?" She said, "Honey, you can't do an MRI. That metal valve will rip right out of your chest!" Thank goodness she was on top of her game that day. I guess the lesson here is to keep talking to the nurses and technicians. They are your fail-safe to a large extent. You just don't have the ability or mental capacity to second-guess everything that's going on. And the doctors don't always know the whole picture. This gets right back to managing the process. If needed, stop, back up, and ask for help.

Several months later, the MRI was reordered. This time Ann checked the facts with her reconstruction surgeon who explained the MRI would be harmless, as the expander (trade name Mentor) was specifically designed to be safe when doing the test. Ann went into the machine quite nervous, but all was well, and the expander was not ripped from her chest.

Nipple Reconstruction & Areola Tattoo—We are now through the reconstruction and all I can say is, "Thank goodness for modern technology and good plastic surgeons." There is life after a mastectomy and, with luck, it won't be lop-sided!

So, you start with the expander, which will grow to truly alpine greatness and will, in the end, cause some discomfort potentially requiring pain medication. But then, drugs are our friend, right? When the expander came out in June 2008 and the permanent implant went in, we were all smiles. A nipple reconstruction took place in September. I was there, and this process was really weird—pulling skin together and creating something from nothing. Unfortunately, the nipple didn't hold, which sometimes happens. Ann didn't want a flat nipple, so our gifted surgeon stitched her up again in December, this time with a much bigger nipple. She chuckled and commented that if she had overdone it in size, she could just decapitate the excess. Interesting concept! In reality, it shrank on its own.

In January 2009, seventeen months after starting down this road, it was time for the final touch—tattooing the areola. Now, if we are honest, there are just certain things a guy should be ignorant about. I think this is one of them! Ann had read an article saying that one of the newest techniques was to have a tattoo artist do the areola versus having it done at a hospital by nurses who don't really specialize in tattoos. So, off we went to Little Vinnie's Tattoos north of Baltimore. Vinnie, according to the article, specialized in this and was a master. Ann insisted I go with her to see Vinny, the areola expert. I'm a staunch believer that tattooing should only be done by Harley riders with a death wish. I was uncomfortable to the extreme. The medical staff could have done this in the hospital, but, by their own admission, they are not experts in the field.

The tat parlor was very clean, and Vinny was a true gentleman! Nonetheless, I've done some bizarre things in my life, but this takes the cake (or at least makes the top five). Sitting in this small room, I watched Vinny touch and rub my beloved's breasts...ARE YOU

KIDDING ME? I couldn't take him out, what would she think? Besides, he was a nice guy. Turns out he has done hundreds of these, many in doctors' offices. Grin and bloody well bear it!

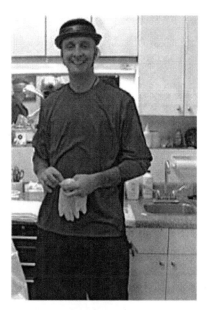

Little Vinnie, the "Master Boobologist."

Vinny, I've thought of myself as a "booboligist" for many years, but I bow in awe and admiration to the "master." You did it, and she looks great! More than great…she looks wonderful!

So there is life after mastectomy. Please enjoy it as much as we do!

CHAPTER 18

Holistic Healing

No system of treatment has a monopoly on curing patients. So when faced with cancer, we figured we should look into options beyond conventional medicine. There seemed to be two schools of thought on this: 1) complementary medicine, and 2) alternative medicine. Both focus on balancing the whole person—physically, mentally and emotionally—with the end result a more holistic healing.

Complementary medicine is defined by non-conventional therapeutic techniques that are used together with traditional medicine (surgery, radiation, chemo, hormone therapy) as an additional "complement." This practice might include acupuncture, massage, Reiki, yoga, visualization, meditation, aromatherapy, journaling, music therapy, and hypnosis, just to name some of the more common choices.

By contrast, alternative medicine is used "in place of" conventional medicine. As such, it is far more controversial and not generally condoned by medical practitioners. An example might be to use a special diet or shark cartilage instead of surgery to combat the cancer.

For many people with breast cancer, both holistic approaches have been shown to help relieve symptoms, ease treatment side-effects, reduce fatigue, reduce stress, improve sleep, and improve quality of life.

Our dear friend Dawna has battled three different kinds of cancer over the past forty years. Each time she elected to do something other than traditional medicine and succeeded in putting the cancer into remission. As she describes it, she has learned to thrive with cancer, not just live with it. So, we knew that alternative approaches can work. However, an important element to success is belief at the deepest level of your being that you can harness the mind/body connection to create healing. Ann just wasn't there. She did, however, have a strong belief that complementary techniques would enhance her well-being, so she went that route.

A number of studies have found that more than 70 percent of breast cancer survivors have used at least one complementary technique. So, for those of you out there who think this is a bunch of rubbish, open your mind and support your partner in trying some new things. She can also apply techniques, like massage, that were previously used for other purposes to battle her breast cancer. This is a pretty personal thing in terms of what fits your needs, belief system, preferences, and style. For more information, log onto www.breastcancer.org . Go to Treatment and Side Effects and then to Complementary & Holistic Medicine. The M.D. Anderson Cancer Center also provides useful information at: www.mdanderson.org/departments/CIMER

The following is a bit on our experience with the complementary practices that Ann tried, though it doesn't begin to cover the options available. Bear in mind, what worked for us, may not work for you.

Reiki—Reiki means "universal life energy." Reiki practitioners believe that energy surrounds and moves through the human body. By moving energy with their hands, practioners balance the flow of energy and stimulate the body's healing abilities. Although there are no scientific studies showing that Reiki cures cancer, there are plenty of people around that believe it helps. Ann's friend Patty regularly performed Reiki on Ann (remotely from Colorado) for several months, from the time of surgery through chemo and beyond. My brother Doug also did some remote Reiki sessions and provided the hands-on treatment when visiting. Ann swears that the Reiki made a big difference in her overall health, energy and her ability to recover from surgery and each chemo treatment.

Journaling—Journaling is creating a written account of events and emotions that you experience. It is sometimes coupled with drawing pictures or images. It's a great way to express thoughts, feelings, ideas, or concerns. Ann started with a traditional written journal, but drawing images seemed to stimulate her more. Then we came up with the idea of this book, with the intent to help others going through this traumatic experience. Whether or not we are successful is probably not relevant in the grand scheme of things, as our hearts were engaged, and it was therapeutic to put our experience into writing. That's what journaling is all about.

Visualization—Sometimes called guided imagery, with this technique a person imagines pictures, sounds, smells, and other sensations associated with reaching a goal. Imagining a certain environment or situation can activate the senses, producing a physical or psychological effect. Studies have shown that visualization can help relieve anxiety, depression, and moodiness in breast cancer patients. Trust me—if she is relieved, you will be too! There are plenty of CDs available that take you through the process, so it might be worthwhile buying one and giving it as a gift for her to try. A variation of this technique that Ann liked was repeating positive affirmations. Friend Patty again jumped into action and made Ann some affirmation cards to stimulate her thinking, but there are numerous books on this subject. Louise Hay is one such author.

Another variation of visualization Ann liked was around "the wearing of the rings." To support her, several friends from around the world each wore a pink ring purchased from the Susan G. Komen Web site. Ann visualized the rings radiating warmth and love. In June 2008, she had a Pink Ring Party. Each woman took off her ring, signed it, and placed it in a beautiful container with a sleeping fairy on top. This was Ann's way of visualizing the cancer at rest. Those who lived elsewhere had a private ceremony and told Ann what they did for closure.

Hypnosis—Hypnosis has been shown to help reduce pain, nausea, vomiting, stress, and anxiety, but you must be open and receptive to the idea of hypnosis for it to work. In Ann's case, she had done some previous past-life regressions through hypnosis. Rather than use hypnosis to reduce symptoms, she tried another past-life regression to see if there might be unresolved conflict she was carrying around that impacted her condition. Frankly, I struggle with this concept a bit. However, I supported her effort. In one of her prior regressions, she found herself as a scullery maid and I was the lord of the manor. We had an affair, but being a true nobleman, I left her for greener pastures. True? Who knows? But we now have changed places, as she is the lady of the manor and I am …?

Music Therapy—Music is medicinal. It can be used to create energy, help you relax, stimulate thinking, and bring about physical/ emotional/ mental release and healing.

In support of our zest to experiment, Dawna sent a CD with chanting. It obviously had worked for her but brought tears to our eyes. Actually, that is an understatement. We put the CD on and lasted about halfway through it. I decided that chanting sucks bigtime. I screamed, "Enough is enough! If this is working for you, I'm leaving the house for a while." Annie said she was struggling a bit, as well. So, out it came. It is amazing; what works for some people does not for others. But, you have to try it all, in some respects. Thankfully, Dawna's husband, Andy Bryner, is a professional pianist who wrote a song for Ann. That was much more our style and very appreciated.

Nutrition—I am not even going to attempt to address this one, as the field is so broad and the application is targeted to the individual. Stories abound of people who have tried, with success, some pretty radical nutrition regimes. For example, we know someone who swears by wheat grass juice. My only advice is to have a conversation with your oncologist about ideas you may be considering, and keep him/her informed as you try new things.

Look, the whole thing about holistic healing is that if you believe in it, it will likely help. The human mind is the most powerful energy source in the world. When it focuses on a solution or belief, things can and do happen—even physical changes. Personally, I tend to be skeptical of some non-traditional healing practices, but I can't dismiss that which many people have experienced. So, if you go down this path, remain open and willing to experiment, but keep the end-game in mind.

CHAPTER 19

The End and A Beginning

I finished the manuscript, or rather, it finished me. I was wiped out. Being a first time author, I didn't realize how exhausting the process would be. Particularly because in writing the Primer, I relived our experience with breast cancer from start to finish. So, when Ann said it needed a conclusion, I came up blank. Perhaps that is what the more experienced authors call writer's block or maybe there is no conclusion per se. Not to be overly dramatic, but this is just a slice out of the timeline of our lives. The good news is the timeline continues.

My original intent had been to provide a brief guide to those who wish to support a partner with breast cancer. But, as I noted early in the book, most of what I included would apply to supporting a person with any type of cancer— not just from the perspective of a spouse or life partner but also as a family member or good friend.

In reliving what we had been through, I realized how naïve we had both been pre-BC. We had family and friends who had gone through breast cancer, as well as other types of cancer and serious illnesses, but we really didn't fully appreciate their experience. I think that's because we provided encouragement and support but stayed on the sidelines, in many respects. In hindsight, there was more we could have done.

I think about my mother who had cancer. I stood by her side and comforted her, but I could have done more. We had a business colleague, only in her thirties, who was diagnosed with a very aggressive and ultimately fatal breast cancer. She often came to mind while Ann was sick. I recalled watching our colleague go from a vibrant, opinionated young woman to a true fighter, frail and bald. Little did we truly understand the significance of her struggle and what we could have done to be more supportive. Knowing what we know now, it is hard not to wish for a few do-overs in life.

We are now at a junction with a new beginning. We know so much more, and our capacity to support others has increased tremendously. Hopefully, you got something from our journey (a summary of which is included in Appendix A) that will help prepare you for yours—whether you need to support your partner or someone else close to you.

There is no magic formula to make it come out right, but I believe you will be on the path to successful support if you do the following:

1. Be loving and caring—there are hundreds of ways to demonstrate this regardless of geographic proximity.
2. Be supportive—think broadly about what this could look like for the individual, given their particular situation. Ask them what they need.
3. Get organized—don't procrastinate or you'll be lost before you know it. (But stay away from the nests they build.)
4. Manage the process—get into your role as a partner, friend, or family member. Don't stand on the sidelines waiting for direction.
5. Never make a decision before it is time—you'll be pressured at times to move forward quickly, but if your gut says to slow down, listen to it.
6. Never solve a problem until it exists—It's natural to jump ahead and try to solve all the "what ifs." However, you have only so much emotional energy. Use it sparingly!
7. Take on additional duties—this is an area where partners, family and friends can shine. Just look around and see what needs to be done. Don't expect the person in need to

ask, as they are already feeling guilty about all you are doing.

8. Encourage a physical regimen—help them get some exercise, even if it's just a short, slow walk. Exercise is good for the body, mind, and soul.

9. Take care of yourself, as well—you can't be effective in supporting someone else if you are not at your best. Be mindful of your whole self physically and emotionally. Get help from others, if needed. That's what friends are for.

10. Never ever forget the end-game—with any serious illness it's about doing everything you can to get better and feeling loved and supported in the process, regardless of the final outcome.

Fortunately, you don't have to be a rocket scientist to make this happen. All you need is a big heart and a willingness to try.

Throughout Ann's recovery, we kept the end-game in sight and our story has a happy ending. Annie is now cancer free, although she'll be taking the hormone therapy pills for years. The health challenges resulted in bringing us even closer together as life partners. On September 4, 2008, we celebrated life and our twenty-fifth wedding anniversary by renewing our marriage vows in a ceremony that had deep emotional significance for both of us. In many ways, this truly felt like the beginning of a brand new relationship. Thanks to good friends Captain Lee and Lady Sher for being a big part of this special event.

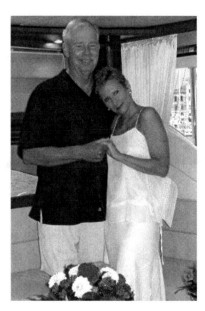

**Our Twenty-fifth Anniversary
recommitment ceremony.**

There is a good news/bad news scenario about all this that I feel obligated to mention. The good news is obvious: cancer free, hair, nails firming up and a hell of a lot less soup on the menu. We are living large!

The bad news? Well, you know all those neat things you did, all the love and attention you gave, and all your hours of sacrifice? They were warranted and justified; hopefully, a successful conclusion was reached. But, you may have opened up Pandora's Box and inadvertently shown sides of yourself that were not previously apparent. Guess what? THEY LIKE IT! OOPS!

"C'mon honey, you can help me with the sheets."

"What? Sheets?"

"Yes, those things you like to sleep on and changed for me a few times while I was sick."

"Yeah, but that was because..."

"Because what? Spit it out!"

"Never mind. Be right there."

"I don't feel like cooking tonight."

"Okay, where would you like to go?"

"I actually don't feel like going out."

"Let's see, you don't feel like cooking, and you want to stay home."

"I knew you would understand."

"Perhaps I should cook dinner tonight."

"Great idea! I'll be in the den reading a book."

"I'm off to get my hair done, and then have lunch with the girls. Be a dear and watch the laundry, would you? I've started everything and there are only three or four more loads. Ciao!"

"But, but, but…" The door slams.

In the final analysis, these are probably small prices to pay, but you can say goodbye to any illusions you had that life will return to what it was. It will be familiar, but it will definitely be different.

Two universal truths come to mind. First, as an old mentor of mine was fond of saying, "No good deed goes unpunished." Second, there are always unintended consequences!

Good luck and best wishes on your journey. Don't forget to celebrate life daily!

APPENDIX A

Our Treatment Timeline: What to Expect and How to Support

Diagnosis & Plan of Attack	Surgery & Treatment	Recuperation & Reconstruction	Follow Up
About 1 1/2 –2 Months	About 6–7 Months	About 7–9 Months	Ongoing
What To Expect —Shock, anger, fear —Being overwhelmed —Emotions a-plenty **Emotional Support** —Be there with body, mind and heart! —Hold hands —Show love & understanding —Don't over play the "what ifs" **Key Activities** —Get 2nd/3rd opinions —Decide medical team —Sort insurance coverage —Understand timeline —Ask lots of questions **Other Ways To Help** —Take notes —Start record of tests, visits, etc. —Be courier for records —Mutually decide who to tell & when —Help communicate **How I Was Feeling** —Shock, anger, fear —Overwhelmed —Desire to 'fix it"	**What To Expect** —Anxiety —Feeling lousy, fatigue —Sense of loss for breast, hair —Chemo brain —Less interest in sex **Emotional Support** —Be there! —Lots of hand holding & love —Insert some humor —Initiate candid talk —<u>Ask</u> what she needs & how to help her **Key Activities** —Attend surgeries —No alone chemos/ radiation —Get support & use it —Create distractions —Get her moving —Manage medical bills —Find nonsexual ways to show intimacy **Other Ways To Help** —Do chores —Grocery shop & cook —Stay out of her nests —Go with the flow for hair, chemo brain, sex —Do the little things (music, clean sheets) **How I Was Feeling** —Worried —Uncertain what to do —Protective	**What To Expect** —Potential pain —Chemo brain lingers —Ups/ downs in energy —Anxious to get back to normal (hair, body) —Uncertainty around intimacy **Emotional Support** —Be there! —Lots of hand holding & love —Insert some humor —Keep communications open —Provide positive reinforcement **Key Activities** —Attend surgeries —Plan outings with friends/family —Encourage increased physical activity —Manage medical bills —Let loose: help her transition to her normal routine **Other Ways To Help** —Continue helping with chores/ cooking —Splurge a bit on hairdresser, nails, etc. —Keep doing the little things **How I Was Feeling** —Sense of optimism —Tired —Empowered	**What To Expect** —Anxiety over next test & BC returning —Renewed desire to live life to fullest —Some side effects from surgery / meds **Emotional Support** —Be there! —Do the follow-up but don't live life around the next test —Understand the fear never leaves **Key Activities** —Enjoy life – plan fun, see the kids —Finalize medical bills —Ensure follow-up happens —As partner, get back to your own routine **Other Ways To Help** —Keep doing some chores/ cooking —Talk about the BC journey —Get involved with support groups **How I Was Feeling** —Light at the end of the tunnel —Gratitude —Triumphant

APPENDIX B

Breast Cancer References

Typically, at the end of a book you find some alphabetized list of references. This is usually a good thing. It does, however, leave the reader with the task of sifting through the information to figure out what might work for them. Therefore, I've added a few editorial comments to try and help with this effort.

The other thing about breast cancer references is that there are a whole lot of them. I could probably include ten pages of these without much sweat. As a matter of fact, when you start this process you'll find it's like peeling a big onion. It seems like there are unlimited options. While this may appeal to a researcher, it's daunting and frustrating when you have decisions to make to get to the end-game.

Finally, almost all references are targeted to women. Very few are specifically male or partner oriented. Listed below are the sources that worked for Ann and me, for one reason or another.

Resources Targeted to Men

Breast Cancer Husband: How To Help Your Wife (and Yourself) Through Diagnosis, Treatment, and Beyond by Marc Silver

Written from a husband's perspective, the book seeks to provide spouses with much needed information on the whole breast cancer journey. Marc interviewed numerous surgeons, oncologists, and breast cancer patients and includes both insights and tips from them. It is long, at about three hundred pages, but if hearing other people's stories will help you, get this one.

For The Women We Love - A Breast Cancer Plan and Caregiver's Guide for Men by Matthew J. Loscalzo with Marc Heyison

    This is a short, easy-to-read caregiver's guide for men. The authors note, and I agree, that it is a no-nonsense navigation and survival guide for men who are committed to being there for the women they love. This book is a highly structured road map that will give you a better understanding of what the patient and caregiver are up against. Marc founded the organization "Men Against Breast Cancer."

Men Against Breast Cancer—The goal of MABC is to educate and empower men to be there for women during and after their battle against breast cancer. **www.menagainstbreastcancer.org**

Other Organizations and Web Sites

American Cancer Society—This is an organization with which we are all familiar. The Web site is a great place to start if you or your loved one has cancer. Information is provided on many types of cancer, including references to other sources to assist your specific needs. www.cancer.org

Breastcancer.org—This site covers a wide range of information on breast cancer: symptoms, diagnosis, treatments, side effects, research, and even includes a chat room. It also provides a good overview of complementary and holistic medicine. This was Ann's "go to" Web site, and she highly recommends it. www.breastcancer.org

Look Good...Feel Better—This is a free non-medical, brand-neutral national public service program founded to help women offset appearance-related changes from cancer treatment. The organization hosts seminars on just what the title says. If you are fighting cancer and dealing with many physical issues, check it out. The Web site also includes information for teens and men who are dealing with the side effects of cancer treatment. www.lookgoodfeelbetter.org

Living Beyond Breast Cancer—Whether you need information on breast cancer treatment, breast cancer recurrence, testing, or side effects, this organization offers a wealth of information. It was originally founded to support women after treatment but now assists women at all stages of diagnosis, treatment and recovery. www.lbbc.org

Live Strong —This is associated with the Lance Armstrong Foundation. As you might guess, it is designed to inspire a winning attitude. It is a particularly good site for young adults with cancer. www.livestrong.org

M.D. Anderson Cancer Center—M. D. Anderson is a world-renowned cancer center located in Houston, Texas. Their Web site includes information on most forms of cancer. Ann used their Web site on complementary and integrative medicine education to help her decide how to integrate such therapies into her care. www.mdanderson.org/departments/CIMER

Susan G. Komen For The Cure—This is another organization with which you are likely familiar. It is the largest source in the world of nonprofit funds dedicated to the fight against breast cancer. The Web site has lots of useful information on breast cancer It also includes details on events with which you may want to be involved, as well as a cool gift shop where you can purchase all sorts of support merchandise This is where the pink rings came from that Ann's friends wore to support her. You really need to take a look at this Web site. www.komen.org

Books

Crazy Sexy Cancer Tips by Kris Carr—If you are looking for inspiration in fighting a cancer battle, this one will do it. Kris was thirty-one years old when she was told she had a very rare vascular cancer affecting the lining of the blood vessels in her lungs and liver. At Stage IV, she wasn't given much hope to live, so she went to work on strengthening her immune system through diet and lifestyle. She delivers a candid and humorous account of her experience, as well as stories from friends that have had cancer. Check out her Web site at www.crazysexycancer.com

Dr. Susan Love's Breast Book by Susan M. Love, M.D.—This is THE reference book on breast cancer. It's not an easy or quick read (very long and technical) but was the best complete resource on breast cancer we found. We did not read it cover to cover, but Ann referred to it frequently to understand various aspects of what she was going through. Dr. Love also has a Web site: www. susanlovemd.org

Health and Healing by Andrew Weil, M.D.— If you want to explore alternative healing practices, this book is a good first step. Written by a doctor, it provides insights on the full spectrum of options, including holistic medicine, homeopathy, osteopathy, Chinese medicine, and others. It will get you thinking about ways to complement traditional medicine approaches.

Navigating Breast Cancer —A Guide for the Newly Diagnosed by Lillie Shockney—This was the first book we were given, and its title describes exactly why it is so useful. This quick, easy read gave us a jump start on what we were dealing with and what to expect (mostly from a woman's perspective). If you are just starting out on the BC journey, get this book.

LaVergne, TN USA
13 January 2010
169963LV00004B/166/P